The Psychiatric Hospitalist

A Career Guide

The Psychiatric Hospitalist

A Career Guide

Edited by

Michael D. Jibson, M.D., Ph.D.

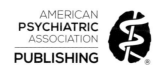

AMERICAN
PSYCHIATRIC
ASSOCIATION
PUBLISHING

If you wish to buy 50 or more copies of the same title, please go to www.appi.org/specialdiscounts for more information.

Copyright © 2022 American Psychiatric Association Publishing

ALL RIGHTS RESERVED

First Edition

Manufactured in the United States of America on acid-free paper
25 24 23 22 21   5 4 3 2 1

American Psychiatric Association Publishing
800 Maine Avenue SW, Suite 900
Washington, DC 20024-2812
www.appi.org

Library of Congress Cataloging-in-Publication Data

Names: Jibson, Michael Dell, 1952- editor. | American Psychiatric Association Publishing, publisher.

Title: The psychiatric hospitalist : a career guide / edited by Michael D. Jibson.

Description: First edition. | Washington, DC : American Psychiatric Association Publishing, [2022] | Includes bibliographical references and index.

Identifiers: LCCN 2021032205 (print) | LCCN 2021032206 (ebook) | ISBN 9781615371389 (paperback ; alk. paper) | ISBN 9781615373871 (ebook)

Subjects: MESH: Hospitalists—organization & administration | Hospitals, Psychiatric—organization & administration. | Psychiatry—methods | Vocational Guidance

Classification: LCC RC439 (print) | LCC RC439 (ebook) | NLM WM 21 | DDC 362.2/1—dc23

LC record available at https://lccn.loc.gov/2021032205

LC ebook record available at https://lccn.loc.gov/2021032206

British Library Cataloguing in Publication Data

A CIP record is available from the British Library.

Contents

PART I
Framework

1 The Hospitalist Model in Psychiatry. 3
Laura Hirshbein, M.D., Ph.D.

2 Inpatient Services 17
Michael D. Jibson, M.D., Ph.D.

3 Consultation-Liaison Psychiatry. 29
Sarah Mohiuddin, M.D.
Wael Shamsedeen, M.D.

PART II
Skill Set

PART III
Clinical Care

PART IV
Special Issues

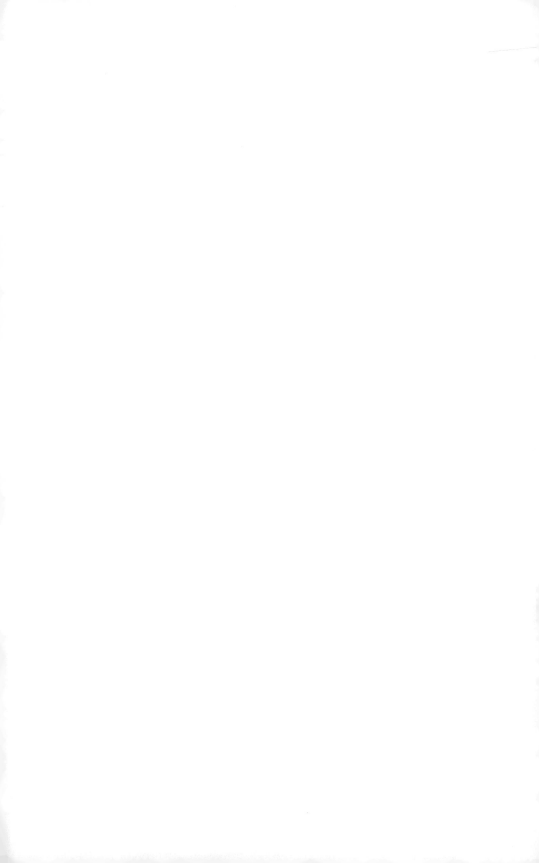

Contributors

Joshua Bess, M.D.
Medical Director, Seattle Neuropsychiatric Treatment Center, Seattle, Washington

Paul R. Borghesani, M.D., Ph.D.
Associate Professor of Psychiatry and Behavioral Sciences, Harborview Medical Center and University of Washington School of Medicine, Seattle, Washington

Katrina Bozada, M.D.
Assistant Professor of Psychiatry, University of Michigan, Ann Arbor, Michigan

Michael Casher, M.D.
Associate Emeritus Professor of Psychiatry, University of Michigan, Ann Arbor, Michigan

Heidi Combs, M.D., M.S.
Professor of Psychiatry and Behavioral Sciences, Harborview Medical Center and University of Washington School of Medicine, Seattle, Washington

Laura Hirshbein, M.D., Ph.D.
Professor of Psychiatry and History, University of Michigan, Ann Arbor, Michigan

Michael D. Jibson, M.D., Ph.D.
Professor of Psychiatry, University of Michigan, Ann Arbor, Michigan

Nasuh Malas, M.D., M.P.H.
Associate Professor of Psychiatry and Pediatrics, University of Michigan, Ann Arbor, Michigan

Stephen Mateka, D.O.
Medical Director, Inspira Bridgeton Child & Adolescent Psychiatry Services, Merchantville, New Jersey

Sarah Mohiuddin, M.D.
Assistant Professor of Psychiatry, University of Michigan, Ann Arbor, Michigan

Heather E. Schultz, M.D., M.P.H.
Assistant Professor of Psychiatry, University of Michigan, Ann Arbor, Michigan

Wael Shamsedeen, M.D.
Assistant Professor of Psychiatry, American University of Beirut Medical Center, Beirut, Lebanon

Ahmad Shobassy, M.D.
Assistant Professor of Psychiatry, University of Michigan, Ann Arbor, Michigan

Bradley Stilger, M.D.
Assistant Professor of Psychiatry, University of Michigan, Ann Arbor, Michigan

Gerald Scott Winder, M.D., M.Sc.
Associate Professor of Psychiatry and Surgery, University of Michigan, Ann Arbor, Michigan

Preface

We are the keepers of hope.

Valerie Barrie, R.N., B.S.N.

Hospitalist psychiatry as a career choice alongside other "intensivist" specialties is still struggling to be given serious consideration. Outside of large multiunit long-term facilities, hospital care in both academic and community settings generally has been envisioned as not quite an afterthought but at least not a core component of clinical work. Traditionally, the community psychiatrist's morning rounds on inpatients otherwise managed by nurses and activity therapists merely opened the day as a task to be handled before the more germane work of the outpatient clinic. The academician's one dreaded month each year when research had to be set aside to satisfy the demands of the department seemed a necessary but unpleasant distraction from the tenure-yielding pursuits of the laboratory. Only recently have we seriously questioned those models.

Three decades ago, I came to the realization that I enjoyed two professional activities above all others—teaching and high-acuity clinical care. Through a fortuitous turn of events, I found my way to the perfect career, with a full clinical load of inpatients and a substantive role in medical education. My satisfaction with those activities has never waned, but the world around me has changed. Much has been written about the decreasing availability, in both beds and hospital days, of hospital-based care, but that is not

the change that I find most interesting. Instead, I am fascinated and gratified by what has happened among the psychiatrists who choose to work in
the hospital setting.

Gradually but steadily, I have been surrounded by a cadre of colleagues
whose professional lives, like mine, never leave the hospital. They are
mostly young, often coming straight from residency or fellowship, sometimes set in their directions and sometimes just trying things out. They have
but one common quality: an interest in the most acute patients, most intense treatments, and most dynamic interactions in the field. As students,
they learned the basics of psychopathology, clarified for them by its most
florid presentations. As residents, they learned the skills of treatment,
guided by the shoulder-to-shoulder tutelage of their faculty. Yet as early career psychiatrists in this seemingly familiar setting, they struggle to navigate the more subtle aspects of this professional path, often without the
benefit of an appropriate mentor.

This book was conceptualized for these newcomers to the field. My fellow authors and I wrote the advice that we would give to a junior colleague
launching a career in hospital-based psychiatry. The result turned out more
generally applicable than that, with insights and recommendations that
even I as an experienced hospitalist find enlightening and refreshing. With
a few exceptions, this book is not about the clinical aspects of hospital care
but rather about the skills and perspectives that allow us to provide that care
and flourish professionally in the process.

It is my hope that armed with these tools, you will find your way
through the myriad challenges, both clinical and practical, that make this
work so daunting. I also hope that this book will convey some of the excite-
ment and satisfaction that come uniquely through the hospital setting. I will
add, just as I do with every student and resident on the first day of their clinical rotations, when their long preparation in the lecture hall and the library
gives way to the moment they can walk through our doors to be part of a
world they had only imagined, "Welcome to the hospital psychiatry service.
This will be an experience like no other."

Michael D. Jibson, M.D., Ph.D.

Acknowledgments

It is with tremendous gratitude
that I acknowledge three types of contributors to this book. First, I am grateful to my coauthors for their great faith and outstanding work in producing their chapters. I appreciate their insights, their efforts to make them accessible to us all, and their patience in the protracted process of publication.

Second, I am grateful to Laura W. Roberts, M.D., M.A., the long-suffering and ever-encouraging editor-in-chief of American Psychiatric Association Publishing. Without her inspired combination of prodding and praise, this project would have foundered on the shoals of my sometimes-flagging efforts.

Third, I feel continued kinship and appreciation for the primary mentors who guided me through the painful days of my inpatient apprenticeship—most notably, C. Peter Rosenbaum, M.D.—who stood beside me in the trenches of my internship day after day, gently reflecting on my efforts in the work we shared and modeling the skills he acquired over a long and distinguished career. I have not forgotten the many conversations we had in the respite of an umbrella-shaded table in the yard outside the inpatient unit in the hinterlands of Stanford Hospital. I am similarly grateful to the staff of the late "flight deck" at the Palo Alto VA Medical Center, where I spent my first few months as an inpatient attending (on the same unit where Ken Kesey had worked 30 years before), who tolerantly guided me into that role. I likewise appreciate my University of Michigan mentors—most notably, John F. Greden, M.D., who as chair took a chance on a not particularly promising young faculty candidate, and Rajiv Tandon, M.D., whose breadth of knowledge, passion for the work, and ceaseless mentoring made my first faculty years a period of unparalleled growth. Finally, I am grateful to the hospital nursing, social work, and activity therapy staff at University of Michigan Hospital who so capably exemplify the highest ideals of professionalism and service, as reflected in the insightful words of Valerie Barrie, R.N., B.S.N., at her (first) retirement. Those words inspire me every day.

PART I
Framework

CHAPTER 1
The Hospitalist Model in Psychiatry

Laura Hirshbein, M.D., Ph.D.

Hospitalist psychiatry is a new name for an old way of doing things in mental health care. If we go back far enough in the history of American psychiatry, all members of the profession were by definition hospitalists—physicians who specialized in the hospital treatment of mentally ill patients. The original name for the American Psychiatric Association was the Association of Medical Superintendents of American Institutions for the Insane. But as outpatient treatment became increasingly favored as the ideal intervention in mental health for those with mild to moderate disorders (neuroses) by the 1940s and after the de-institutionalization movement in the 1960s (psychoses), hospital care of mentally ill patients received relatively little positive attention.

The trend until fairly recently was to manage the need for inpatient care—now measured in days to weeks—with either faculty who rotated for a period of time at an academic hospital or private psychiatrists who managed both a clinic and an inpatient caseload. This model was based on the traditional method used by general medicine and surgery services throughout the United States. Although those in practice could avoid hospital activity if they so desired, many inside and outside academia spent some of their time taking care of acutely ill patients in the hospital. In some hospitals, psychiatrists picked up extra work when they were assigned the task of seeing patients with psychiatric problems on medical or surgical floors in consultation with their providers or of doing consultations in the emergency department.

In recent years, some psychiatrists have been following a model developed within medicine: the hospitalist system. Instead of having academic faculty rotate on hospital services for a month or two during the year or having private practice physicians see patients in the office during one part of the day and then travel to the hospital to complete rounds on patients there, some hospitals have moved toward having dedicated physician staffs located only within the hospital who care for all patients there. For medical and surgical teams, this has made a lot of sense. Hospital patient populations have been getting progressively sicker, and the medical knowledge needed to treat them has become more specialized. It has seemed less reasonable, for example, for a physician who routinely managed blood pressure in ambulatory patients to be expected—for 1 month a year—to handle hypertensive crisis in an intensive care unit patient.

Not only have medical specialists begun to differentiate based on their ability to take care of sick patients in the hospital but also hospitalist teams have increasingly mobilized to take care of shortages in house officer workforces. Although hospitals were once entirely dependent on training physicians for labor, the expansion of hospitals (without a commensurate increase in training program numbers), as well as changes in what is reimbursable by insurance by level of training and work hours restrictions for residents, have led to a reduced reliance on trainees. Instead, hospitals are using mid-level providers (physician assistants and nurse practitioners) and hospital-based attendings to staff the units.

The hospitalist model in psychiatry has not yet seemed as obvious a solution to either practice challenges or trainee shortages and has been slower to take hold within the profession. For many in the field, psychiatric hospitals are uncomfortable reminders of a history of long-term institutionalization. Although what we do now bears little resemblance to the old state hospital system, some of the public perception of psychiatric institutions can be negative. In addition, some places have so few psychiatrists that there is an insufficient critical mass of professionals to staff a hospital. And much of the professional identity of psychiatrists has been oriented around long-term relationships with patients.

However, it makes sense to think about hospital-based psychiatry. The hospital is where the sickest patients get care. For psychiatric patients, that means the acutely agitated and possibly violent patients who go to the emergency department, the patients who have seriously harmed themselves and need treatment in a medical setting, and those who are so intent on taking their own lives that they need to be on a locked inpatient unit. Many psychiatrists are uncomfortable with this level of intensity, but these patients' problems cannot be contained within the traditional office practice structure. Even for those psychiatrists who try to split their time between an office and the hospital, certain things (such as the need to emergently medicate a patient or authorize restraints) usually require a provider to be present in the hospital at unpredictable times.

The hospital is not a setting suited to everyone. Some of us immerse ourselves in the hospital because it is a key site for residency education training. All psychiatry residents need to show competency in inpatient, emergency, and consultation-liaison psychiatry, and these settings provide rich opportunities to interact with trainees. Others of us enjoy the team aspects of hospital-based work—collaborating with nurses, social workers, activity therapists, and other medical staff to take care of seriously ill patients. And some of us find that the hospital is the most exciting, dynamic environment in which to confront the most acute patient challenges and take the opportunity to make an immediate and visible difference in patients' lives. But whatever reason you choose for focusing your professional efforts in the hospital, hospital-based psychiatry definitely has advantages and challenges.

Structure of Hospitalist Psychiatry Services

The critical element of hospitalist psychiatry is to have psychiatrists whose primary clinical assignment is the hospital. The core of the model is to have a cadre of specialists who dedicate time and expertise to the specific challenges that arise within the hospital setting. For most hospitals, the bulk of the need is based around the psychiatric inpatient unit. Within this model, the expectation is that psychiatrists be present much of the time on or near the unit (at least during the day) to see patients, be available in case of urgent situations, and engage regularly with the team. A hospitalist psychiatrist could easily be academic. The difference in terms of time management for academic hospital psychiatrists is that they take turns (in blocks of weeks or months) staffing the hospital services with the off-service time devoted to academic endeavors.

The other possible locations within the hospital that benefit from a hospital-based psychiatrist are the emergency department and the consultation-liaison service for medical-surgical patients. Emergency departments are increasingly inundated with patients with substance use disorders and mental health disorders and are struggling to find ways to effectively triage and provide treatment. Some hospitals have more or less specialized psychiatric or behavioral health emergency spaces. The Psychiatric Emergency Services model is used in some locations to allow for a concentrated effort of nurses, social workers, and psychiatrists to better assess patients with behavioral health issues apart from the other kinds of chaos in medical emergency departments. This has been shown to decrease the boarding time in medical emergency departments.

Even without that specialized space, psychiatric hospitalists who can be mobilized in the emergency department can help make better informed decisions about the boundaries between mental and physical health issues, as well as appropriate disposition of patients with psychiatric symptoms. In a similar way, hospital-based psychiatrists can work with medical and surgical teams in a general hospital to provide expertise and support for the complex interactions between medical illness and psychiatric symptoms. Common issues such as delirium, care of a patient following a suicide attempt, and strong emotional reactions to major medical problems are all areas in which consulting psychiatrists who are familiar with the environment of the hospital can be an asset.

Advantages of the Hospitalist Model

Vignette

Dr. M had a 1-month rotation on the inpatient unit of his academic hospital. He was a busy researcher with an erratic schedule, and staff could not predict when he would arrive on the unit. When he was there, he seemed to be preoccupied by the combination of his research and clinical load. He was kind to the patients, but the staff did not feel comfortable telling him things. When one of his patients was getting ready for discharge, the wife of the patient confided to the patient's nurse that she was worried that the patient was lying to the staff about being safe outside the hospital. The nurse tried to find Dr. M to tell him this concern but was unable to locate him until shortly before the patient left. She cautiously offered the wife's concern to Dr. M, but he brushed it off and said that he was confident in his assessment of the patient. A few days later, the staff found out that the patient had gone into the woods and shot himself.

Communication and Teamwork

In acute psychiatric settings, clear communication is essential. Although electronic health records have made the issue of legibility less of a problem, most hospital charting fails to convey the richness and complexity of a patient's presentation and situation. Communication with patients requires face-to-face time, and team interactions are more meaningful when they are conducted in person rather than on the telephone or through the chart. Yes, it is possible to determine when a patient receives medications, how many hours he slept, or his latest vital signs through a chart. But a qualitative difference is seen when the opportunity exists to engage in person. In a team, physicians can learn from the different disciplines: nurses know when and why patients refuse medications or take as-needed medications, activity therapists can report on how patients are functioning in tasks and interacting with others, and social workers communicate with families about their concerns. All of this information is needed to ensure that the patient gets the right treatment and is safely discharged.

Although physicians may or may not be devoted full time to the hospital, the rest of the staff at a hospital generally is. Although physicians' prescriptions determine what kinds of medications the patient may receive or what other major intervention will occur (such as electroconvulsive therapy [ECT]), nurses, activity therapists, and social workers are the ones who spend the bulk of the time with patients. They are also the ones to whom patients and families are more likely to confide thoughts and concerns. A physician who is seldom available or who is not well known to the rest of the staff may not hear about a concern either because he or she is not around or because staff might not feel comfortable communicating that concern. Nurses, social workers, patient care workers, and activity therapists often have good instincts and observational skills. Their assessment of patients' progress (or lack of progress) is important in understanding what interventions still need to be done and when a patient is getting close to discharge. A hospitalist psychiatrist who builds relationships with the team and is more accessible will be in a position—both physically and interpersonally—to get needed information.

Physicians will learn more when they know (and are known by) their teams, and teams will be better able to take direction from familiar physicians. Teams function best with mutual trust. If the rest of the team does not really know a physician, the nurses might unintentionally convey skepticism to patients about the treatment intervention, or the social workers might find themselves in a position of allying with families against the treating physician. There might be delays in physician orders being carried out if the orders are not understood or if the orders are not appropriate for the setting (because of lack of knowledge of the physician). Hospitalist psychiatrists can build trusting relationships with their teams that involve clear communication both internally and externally and also result in clarity of the treatment plans with patients and families.

Consistency, Expertise, and Comfort With Acuity

Consistency is also important, especially for trainees. Psychiatry as a field can be fraught with disagreements in management of some conditions. A patient with mood swings on an hourly basis, who also describes interpersonal chaos, chronic feelings of emptiness, and patterns of self-harm behaviors, might be diagnosed by some psychiatrists as having bipolar disorder and others as experiencing the symptoms of borderline personality disorder. Whatever the merits of either side, trainees need to learn from faculty how to manage patients with symptoms. It is disruptive to trainees—and poor patient care—to have faculty rotate through inpatient settings with wildly different approaches to problem solving and patient presentation. If trainees are assigned to the hospital for up to a year at a time, they could experience a great deal of turmoil with rotating attendings. A smaller cadre of dedicated hospitalist psychiatrists allows more consistency of approach (while permitting individual differences in style or team interaction) to help keep trainees from lurching from one intervention style to another. Furthermore, hospitalist psychiatrists can more easily engage trainees in decision-making (because they are already fully immersed in the environment) and bedside teaching and other educational efforts.

Trainees sometimes experience inconsistent messages from faculty because clinicians have different levels of comfort with acutely ill patients. A psychiatrist who works primarily with depressed patients in an ambulatory setting might not know how to treat a patient with chronic schizophrenia who at baseline is somewhat disorganized and hears voices. The trainee who is attempting to manage this patient might hear from this faculty member that the patient needs to remain in the hospital because of the psychosis, whereas a psychiatrist who works regularly with the chronically mentally ill might have a better understanding that such patients can be supported in the community even when they have symptoms. On a consultation service, a faculty member who has comfort with how to assess suicidal patients might approach a patient with chronic suicidal ideation and self-injurious behavior differently from a faculty member who seldom encounters patients talking about suicide.

In most cases, comfort level develops in parallel with expertise based on experience with many similar cases informed by familiarity with available clinical evidence and consensus guidelines of recognized authorities in the field. This level of engagement facilitates the development of pattern recognition and intuitive understanding that constitutes mastery of any endeavor. Patients benefit from care that is provided by experienced clinicians working in an environment in which they are familiar with the diagnoses, treatments, and other issues they regularly encounter. Hospital-based care is more than just high-level outpatient care. The approaches to diagnosis and treatment; expectations of patients, family, and team members; resources available; and limitations are all unique to the hospital setting and are best handled by those with the most experience and skill with this level of care.

Efficiency

One of the biggest challenges in health care today is the lack of resources, in terms of both space and time and reimbursement. A well-documented benefit of hospitalist medicine is that the model increases efficiency for both admissions to and discharges from the hospital. Psychiatry faces its own problems with regard to throughput at the hospital. Scheduling outpatient appointments is often difficult, and hospital beds are often full. Insurance reimbursement rates are low, and insurance companies are increasingly insisting on rapid transition from hospital to outpatient care. In that setting, a hospital system needs to be as efficient as possible to appropriately and safely move patients from one level of care to another. A physician in the emergency department who is not familiar with psychiatric patients might decide that someone who engages in chronic self-injurious behavior is attempting suicide and needs to be hospitalized, whereas a hospital-based psychiatrist could see the same patient and understand that he would benefit most from a return to his outpatient team that is working with him on dialectical behavior therapy techniques. A rounding faculty member on an inpatient unit who does not know the community resources might be hesitant to discharge a patient to an outpatient team that will follow her. If emergency physicians fill up the scarce psychiatric hospital beds, or if occasional hospital faculty are not comfortable discharging patients, it will become even harder to move patients out of emergency departments, through hospital care, and back to the community.

Not only do psychiatrists who are more comfortable and familiar with acutely ill patients practice in a more efficient manner, but also it becomes easier to deal with insurance issues. As anyone who has worked on an inpatient unit knows, insurance companies are becoming increasingly stingy with authorizations for both admission and continued stays. There is an art to learning to communicate what we are seeing with patients to insurance companies to help them understand how we are trying to help their members. Now that danger to self or others is the major criterion for hospitalization, stating that a patient is still suicidal is not sufficient to obtain authorization. Insurance companies have started to ask more pointed questions such as whether the patient has a plan or an intent to kill himself or herself. It takes practice—and coaching—to convey concerns about patients to the entities that pay for care.

Some psychiatric services such as ECT are more efficient when managed through a hospitalist model. Although many patients can receive ECT treatments when they are living at home, the ECT treatment itself requires a brief staff check-in with a patient, general anesthesia, and recovery time. In many ways, it works much like an outpatient surgery. Within a hospital, an ECT psychiatrist has access to anesthesiology and nurse anesthetists, as well as medical backup in case of a medically unstable patient. An ECT team within a hospitalist model also can easily include inpatients from the psychiatric unit, as well as patients on the medical or surgical services who might benefit from the treatment.

Challenges of the Hospitalist Model

Vignette

Ms. C, a 36-year-old woman with a history of schizophrenia, was hospitalized because of worsening psychotic symptoms, agitation, and aggression toward others in the context of medication noncompliance. The hospital psychiatrist went to court to have Ms. C committed for hospitalization followed by an outpatient treatment order. She continued to insist that she did not need medications but was given a long-acting injectable form of an antipsychotic. The outpatient provider who saw Ms. C after the hospitalization did not get a verbal handoff from the inpatient team, and the discharge summary from the hospital did not mention that Ms. C was receiving court-ordered treatment. When Ms. C told the outpatient doctor that she did not want medication, he did not renew the antipsychotic. Within a few weeks, Ms. C was acutely disorganized and aggressive and required rehospitalization.

Discontinuity in Treatment

When the hospitalist model was first implemented within medicine services in hospitals in the 1990s, the question was raised about how a patient might respond to the discontinuity in care. The assumption was that the hospitalist model was substituting a stranger—the specialized hospital physician—for the patient's physician from the clinic. Concerns were also raised about whether physicians who were attuned to the fiscal and regulatory realities of the hospital would be sufficiently attentive to the needs of the patient. Those issues have been mostly resolved within medical services that use a hospitalist model. But how much are they concerns for hospitalist psychiatrists?

No systematic evidence is available on discontinuity in treatment for psychiatric patients. Many fewer patients are likely in established care relationships with a psychiatrist when they have a crisis that requires psychiatric hospitalization. Patients within the community mental health system are more likely to have episodes of instability, but their treatment teams have been designed to focus on outpatient services rather than inpatient care. For patients who present because of acute substance use issues, the challenge is getting them to engage with any type of provider. Because many outpatient psychiatrists do not have stable, long-term patient populations, relatively few patients would be significantly affected by the discontinuity of a hospitalist psychiatrist.

The potential for hospitalist psychiatrists' divided loyalty to fiscal issues and patient care is harder to assess. Part of the issue is that the purpose of psychiatric hospitalization has changed so much over the past few decades that hospital providers may be more affected by their own experience of the value of the hospital stay than by either what the patient wants or what the insurance company will reimburse. When hospital stays were still measured in months, providers could anticipate that a patient could recover from an episode of depression in the hospital. Today, there is only time to start an antidepressant, make sure a patient is no longer suicidal, and discharge to outpatient care. The reality is that insurance reimbursement for psychiatric hospitalization is limited regardless of where a psychiatrist spends most of his or her time.

Handoffs

Although communication, teamwork, consistency, and efficiency are major advantages within a hospitalist model, there are definitely challenges. One of the most frequently documented concerns is the problem with handoffs to the next level of care provider. All of the rich, important interpersonal interactions that are so helpful in working with patients on inpatient teams would also be helpful in transitioning patients from inpatient to outpatient care, but those interactions are much harder to arrange. In an ideal situation, the inpatient team would know exactly where a discharged patient is headed and would be able to give a verbal handoff to the receiving provider. That ideal often goes unrealized. Some patients do not have established providers before hospitalization. In that context, it is difficult to introduce the patient and his or her issues to a new provider (if he or she could even be reached). Sometimes patients will be engaged in split treatment after discharge and will see a therapist right away while a primary care physician manages medications. Primary care physicians are often hard to reach, and it is not obvious in those cases how much detail to share or what recommendations to make for ongoing care.

Not only is it highly variable in terms of who will be seeing a patient after discharge, but also the timing of the handoff becomes complicated. Discharges have to be managed efficiently, and sometimes inpatient teams do not find out who a patient will be seeing until shortly before he or she leaves the hospital. Trying to reach outpatient providers who have busy clinic schedules is often time-consuming. If a hospital psychiatrist leaves a message for an outpatient psychiatrist about a discharging patient, the receiving physician might not be able to return the call for a few days. In the intervening time, the hospitalist psychiatrist, who has a constantly changing patient population, might lose track of details of an already-discharged patient.

Written handoffs often lack clear information. Regulations on information that has to be conveyed to third-party payers and metrics for quality sometimes mean that discharge summaries are geared toward reimbursement rather than conveying clear information. Accomplishing both with a discharge summary is certainly possible. However, there is a definite art to creating a written handoff that helps an outside provider understand what the patient was like before hospitalization, what happened during the hospital stay, and what the expectation is for treatment following discharge. Of course, the goal of a training program is to teach that art. But training programs have so much to teach residents in terms of patient care that writing discharge summaries seldom gets sustained attention, and physicians vary in their ability to communicate through medical records. The ideal, which requires practice, is to have both written and verbal communication in patient handoffs. This topic is addressed in detail in Chapter 12, "Transitions in Care, Documentation, and Interdisciplinary Communication."

Short-Term Perspective

Another disadvantage of a hospitalist model is that hospital-based psychiatrists can focus so much on acute issues and management in the structured setting that they can lose sight of how patients need to function in their outside lives. This can affect how hospital psychiatrists prescribe medication, for example. In the hospital, it does not matter whether a patient takes a medication three times a day or once—a nurse is available to dispense it. At home, however, it is seldom realistic to expect that patients will administer their own medications with the same thoroughness. Medication selection is also more complicated in a transition to outpatient care. Hospital formularies usually do not make distinctions between levels of cost for medications; either the hospital will allow providers to prescribe medications or they will not. But the medications that are covered and available in the hospital are not necessarily the ones covered by a patient's outpatient pharmacy benefit (if the patient even has one). Patients sometimes have an unpleasant surprise when they go to pick up their discharge prescriptions and discover that the medications they received in the hospital are extremely expensive when they leave.

The short-term perspective is important for hospital psychiatrists. It is critical to be able to focus on the here-and-now and not to become overwhelmed with questions about how the patient might manage long-term problems such as the possible need for disability benefits or a move into assisted living. But the patients who cycle through the hospital do have to worry about these things. It can be overwhelming for patients whose problems started long before the hospital, and will extend long after they are discharged, to be rushed through the hospital process without being able to address some of those issues. During hospitalization, clinicians sometimes miss important details about how patients live their lives.

One way to address this focused perspective of the hospital is to emphasize to patients that we can only address a small part of their lives during the hospital stay. For patients who experienced hospital care decades ago, this will mean managing their expectations to emphasize the change from the past. Other ways of addressing the hospital perspective are to have activity groups that discuss longer-term life issues such as work and leisure. Good collaboration with pharmacists can help with thinking about how patients take medications in the real world and which medications are covered by their insurance.

General Service Issues in Hospital Care

Hospital care, for better or worse, is tightly choreographed and regulated. The presence of multiple different disciplines with their own work and training requirements, as well as third-party payer structures and regulations on the federal, state, and local level, means that hospitals are complicated places in which to work. From the hospital perspective, it does not matter whether physicians work in a hospitalist model or on a drop-in basis—the rules are the same. But the rules are complicated and can be overwhelming to people who are not familiar with them. A good hospital administration system can be invaluable in helping physicians navigate these challenges.

Staffing for Fluctuating Demand

Staffing a hospital service is more complicated than managing outpatient appointments. Hospital emergency services cannot control (or sometimes even predict) the volume of patients who cycle through at any given time. Emergency services likely will be either overstaffed, which can be expensive, or understaffed, which can lead to increased risk when managing acutely psychiatrically ill patients. Consultation services on medical and surgical units can also fluctuate in terms of need. Sometimes medical providers are easily able to manage the emotional or behavioral issues that arise in their patients, but sometimes they ask for more help or they have more patients with major psychiatric problems (such as suicide attempts). It is somewhat more predictable to staff an inpatient psychiatric service, but the length of stay of patients can vary to a large extent, which leads to variable levels of work.

An ideal hospitalist model would have a cadre of psychiatrists who could staff any of the possible areas as demand fluctuated. The overlap in skills between emergency consultation and medical and surgical consultation is extensive, and emergencies drive inpatient admissions. Here again, the advantage of a hospitalist model is that physicians can be deployed when they are needed. An inpatient unit that varies in size based on the availability of its physicians will be less efficient and run the risk of losing resources needed to run the other essential parts of the unit (such as nursing staff and activity therapy).

Legal Issues

All states now have some kind of system of rules to protect patients' rights, specifically around the circumstances in which patients can be kept on locked inpatient psychiatric units and given treatment against their will. Whether or not current psychiatrists appreciate the resulting processes, the states' mental health legal procedures were enacted in response to decades of physician carelessness and what appeared to be patient abuses within long-stay hospitals. Physicians who practice in hospital settings should be aware of the rules that operate within their state regarding inpatient commitment. Some inpatient psychiatrists will need to testify before probate judges about their patients' need for treatment. Court processes can be important to help with residency training, but it is ideal to have some specialized help or guidance from the court for psychiatrists to learn the correct methods of interaction in that setting. Legal issues are discussed in detail in Chapter 14, "Legal and Ethical Issues."

Insurance Issues

Most insurance companies require a physician or social work evaluation to authorize an inpatient admission. The requirements to justify authorization can vary somewhat depending on the insurance company. Some are stricter about demanding that a patient articulate a clear plan and intent for suicide prior to authorizing hospitalization. Others are more willing to understand that sometimes a patient has failed outpatient management and needs a higher level of care. Hospitals must have a staff or system to manage the myriad insurance requirements to ensure that authorization is obtained and to make it clear to the psychiatrist what level of detail in documentation or telephone communication is necessary.

After the initial authorization, most insurance companies require hospitals to demonstrate that patients still meet criteria for continued stay. Again, some companies want hospitals to document that patients are still suicidal with a plan; they might deny continued authorization if a patient is still having suicidal thoughts but no active plan. Some companies move quickly toward a peer review process in which a physician contracted by the insurance company speaks to a hospital psychiatrist about why the patient is still in the hospital. Once again, it is critical for a system to be in place to help the hospital psychiatrists document in the most effective way possible and to facilitate the peer-to-peer review requests that occur.

Regulation

Hospitals are tightly regulated places to work. The Joint Commission, the regulatory body that accredits most hospitals in the United States, has thousands of rules and regulations about what is allowed, what is required, and what is permissible to show that a hospital is meeting an acceptable standard of care. The rules not only are complex but also continue to change. The Joint Commission's rules are enforced by the Centers for Medicare and Medicaid Services, which will withhold payment to hospitals for government insurance programs if hospitals fail to meet specific standards. Although the full management of regulatory requirements necessitates a specific person or an office within a hospital because of the complexity, hospital psychiatrists need to have a basic understanding of how the regulations affect patient care.

KEY POINTS

- Care for high-acuity psychiatric patients remains the domain of hospital-based services, which are best equipped to safely and effectively address high-risk issues such as active suicidality, acute agitation, delirium, and mania.

- The hospitalist model of care exchanges the benefits of a long-term relationship with the patient for those of efficiency, improved teamwork, and higher-level expertise during periods of acute illness.

- The psychiatric hospitalist is able to acquire extensive experience, high comfort level, and specialized knowledge in the acute-care setting to best serve this patient population.

- Familiarity with legal procedures, regulatory issues, and payer expectations is essential.

- Challenges include discontinuity of care and handoff issues both within the hospital and during transitions in care.

- The hospitalist model requires a specific organization of physician schedules, reimbursement system, and administrative infrastructure to function effectively.

CHAPTER 2
Inpatient Services

Michael D. Jibson, M.D., Ph.D.

Inpatient units are the backbone of hospital-based psychiatric care, providing the only venue with sustained, high-intensity mental health services at the level required to address the most acute and severe symptoms. Although sometimes reduced to high-security settings with the sole function of maintaining safety for a suicidal or agitated patient, a properly focused and staffed inpatient unit is ideally suited to address other issues that cannot be fully assessed or treated in less intense settings.

Essential Functions

Safety

As with all clinical care, your highest priority is to ensure the safety of your patient and others nearby. Assess the situation promptly to determine whether the patient is agitated or otherwise an immediate threat. Rate the level of acuity based on information from the transferring service, collateral contacts with family or friends, available records, your initial observations, and your intake evaluation. Ensure that appropriate staffing is available and informed of the level of risk. Limit the patient's access to potentially dangerous items, such as telephone cords, bathroom fixtures, silverware, recreation equipment, and nonessential personal belongings, until staff are confident that the risk of harm is low. Review safety issues with the treatment team daily (see Chapter 16, "Patient Safety").

Evaluation

Evaluate each patient to clarify the nature and extent of the admitting problem, create a differential diagnosis, formulate the case, and begin to construct a treatment plan. The initial evaluation is a first attempt to construct a hypothesis regarding each of these issues, and all will be revised over the course of the patient's stay. In a more generous age (i.e., early in my career), it was not only permissible but also expected that no action would be taken during the first few days of a patient's hospital admission, to allow the staff to observe the full spectrum of the patient's symptoms and to allow the structure and support of the unit to aid the process of recovery. In today's cost-driven environment, such a process is rarely tolerated, and treatment is expected to begin within hours of the patient's arrival. This reality makes the initial assessment all the more important for the hospital course. (For a more thorough review of the evaluation process, see Chapter 8, "Initial Assessment and Treatment Planning.")

Clarify the Problem

Psychiatric diagnoses alone do not require hospitalization. The large majority of individuals with any particular diagnosis did not find their way into your emergency department or onto your inpatient unit. Instead, people are admitted because of a specific type and intensity of problem. Make sure that you understand and address that problem and its underlying causes. A process akin to the "root cause analysis" of adverse event reviews may be appropriate. A suicidal patient simply may be responding to the distress of severe depression but also may be facing real-world losses, intractable challenges, or dilemmas that appear insoluble. Identification of these deeper causes will allow you to better understand the context of the presenting problem and may open additional avenues of intervention.

Vignette

Emily was a freshman at a prestigious university to which she had aspired since childhood. As the end of her first semester approached, she was overwhelmed by impending deadlines for papers she had not yet begun, readings not finished, and final examinations looming. Distraught by the inevitable humiliation of staying and failing her classes or abandoning school to return home and admit that she was not equal to the challenge, she was plucked from a bridge by police alerted to her suicide plan by a roommate who returned early from a party to find her suicide note. In the emergency department, she spoke only of her depression and hopelessness. Once safely housed on the inpatient unit, Emily disclosed her dilemma, triggering a call to the dean's office and intervention with her professors to adjust her schedule and provide her with academic as well as emotional support. Her suicidality and depression quickly resolved.

Make a Diagnosis

Although some interventions will address admitting problems directly, most will target underlying disorders. It is essential, therefore, to determine what each individual's pattern of symptoms is telling you about the neurobiological, psychological, and interpersonal dysfunction that is in play. We do not make diagnoses to label or judge people, nor do we presume to dictate to society what beliefs and behaviors are acceptable and which ones are not. In the absence of direct probes into the individual brain to observe pathology in the style of our cardiology or orthopedic colleagues, we listen to our patients' stories and compare them with the central elements and confirmatory lists of symptoms we find in our professional literature. When we see a close parallel, we offer a diagnosis. This serves a variety of purposes, but one of the most important is to guide treatment, making our diagnoses less about being right or wrong than about being useful or not useful. Fundamentally, the purpose of this process is to help us surmise what is happening in the brain and which interventions may help.

Pharmacological Interventions

Medications are second in importance only to the overall structure of the inpatient unit in the treatment of acute disorders. Despite the limited indications and mechanisms of available medications, they are often useful, even critical, in the acute treatment of most psychiatric disorders.

Medication selection begins with a determination of what class of drug is most appropriate. Fundamentally, only five tools are available in the psychopharmacopoeia: antidepressants, antipsychotics, mood stabilizers, sedative-hypnotics, and stimulants. This realization will greatly simplify initial treatment planning, in that it is only necessary to determine which of these indications is most appropriate for your patient. The selection of a specific drug from within the chosen class is usually given more attention than the comparative data between drugs merit. Differences in efficacy, if they exist, are minor and are far outweighed by the unpredictable response of individuals to specific medications. Side effects and costs are more substantive bases for selection, but the former are as difficult to anticipate for single patients as is effectiveness. Your expertise in this area has less to do with selecting the correct drug on the first try than with knowing what the early signs of response and lack of response to different agents look like and exercising appropriate judgment with regard to when to continue the same treatment and when to make a change. Remember that total dose and duration of treatment are more important factors than drug selection in most treatment plans. This topic is addressed further in Chapter 10, "Guidelines, Algorithms, and Order Sets."

Psychosocial Treatment

The inpatient unit has an additional compelling advantage over other treatment settings in that patients are available for hours every day to participate in a variety of therapeutic activities, some obviously therapeutic in nature and some of more subtle benefit.

Psychotherapy

Psychotherapy modalities appropriate to an acute care service include cognitive-behavioral therapy, dialectical behavior therapy, anger management, and other variants that share a practical, here-and-now approach that can be presented in group settings and that patients can begin to apply immediately. Group therapies have the advantages of efficiency and engagement of peer support. Written materials that clarify, reinforce, and aid subsequent recall of principles presented are a useful addition.

Individual psychotherapy is more variable in its practicality and usefulness. Supportive interventions, especially early in treatment, are frequently helpful. Motivational interviewing can be a critical tool for patients ambivalent about moving forward. Exploratory therapies are occasionally helpful but not without risk. There is rarely time to fully explore early life events and their consequences outside of specialty programs designed for such work. The advisability of opening wounds that might otherwise heal satisfactorily is not always clear and best left to longer-term treatments that will be available after hospitalization.

Activity-Based Therapies

Activity-based therapies encourage physical activity, artistic pursuits, social engagement, distraction, and self-care. Aside from filling long hours in a restricted environment, they lend legitimacy to the use of such activities to relieve the tortured ruminations that accompany so many acute psychiatric conditions. Equally important, they are the best predictor of a patient's capacity for independent and social functioning after discharge. A skilled therapist not only notes (and documents) that a patient participated in a card game with peers but also observes how readily that patient learned the rules of the game, what level of strategy was used, what peer interactions looked like, and how frustrations were handled.

Electroconvulsive and Other Procedural Treatments

The availability of electroconvulsive therapy (ECT) is critical to an inpatient unit, ensuring that the most severely ill patients will get timely access to this intervention. This safe and effective treatment remains deeply stigmatized, largely through misleading portrayals in the media, which may require you to educate patients and families to the nature, side effects, and outcomes involved. Even if you are not credentialed to perform the procedure, you will need to be conversant with these issues as you work with your patients to find the most effective approach to depression, catatonia, bipolar disorder, and other diagnoses. Other procedural interventions, such as transcranial magnetic stimulation, vagus nerve stimulation, and ketamine infusion are more often outpatient treatments but may appropriately be done in the inpatient setting. ECT and other procedural interventions are treated in more detail in Chapter 9, "Diagnostic and Treatment Modalities."

Discharge Management

For acute care inpatient units, all treatment should include preparation for discharge. Rather than thinking of the hospital as the locus of definitive treatment and outpatient care simply as follow-up, conceptualize the inpatient unit as a brief disruption in an ongoing course of outpatient care, which is the actual venue for long-term gains. Check in with the outpatient care provider regularly and make sure that therapy being started in the hospital is consistent with the longitudinal outpatient plan. Keep in mind the setting to which the patient will be transitioning, the level of acuity he or she can handle, and the services they offer. Make sure that the patient will have access to any medications you consider starting. Coordinate discharge as a handoff between providers rather than just an end to your involvement in care.

Documentation

The proliferation of medical record requirements has become one of the great challenges of modern medicine, even leading a significant number of physicians to cite it as a major factor in job dissatisfaction and burnout. The advent of electronic medical records, initially touted as harbingers of efficient and effective means to manage large amounts of information, has instead created massive volumes of repetitive and uninformative records, filled with the "white noise" of prewritten phrases and paragraphs, while demanding tedious and time-consuming note writing that contributes little to patient care. The key to survival in the age of the electronic medical record, is to learn to use its advantages without falling prey to its many blind alleys and sinkholes. A few simple rules will serve you well in this regard.

Write to Your Audience

Before beginning a note, reflect on who will be reading it and what you want to communicate to them. First, think about what you want to remember about today's clinical encounter when you return to the record tomorrow, at discharge, or months from now. Document critical observations that are in flux, including key symptoms, new problems, side effects, and patient concerns. Be clear about what changes in treatment you made and the reasons for those decisions. Consider the needs of other team members who depend on your input for their own treatment decisions, including nurses, activity therapists, and social workers. Communicate clearly your priorities in treatment and explain your reasoning. Make clear to payers why your patient is still hospitalized, what clinical services you provided, and why they were necessary. Develop a realistic sense of what issues need to be recorded for legal purposes, such as safety assessments and informed consent.

Write Well

It is no more difficult to write clear, grammatical, and succinct notes than it is to create sloppy, rambling, and incoherent ones; the difference is simply one of practice and attention. In narratives, write in sentences, with a subject, a verb, and appropriate articles. State things directly rather than circuitously. Avoid service-specific abbreviations that will not be easily understood outside your immediate setting. PTSD, ADHD, ECT, OCD, and CBT are widely and quickly understood; GAD, SI, AVH, PI, SIMD, and SIB are not. Avoid repetition; try to say things once in each note, in the most logical place. Use the initial or interval history to write a qualitative description of events and symptoms. Use the mental status examination to give a quantitative (e.g., 0–10 rating) or comparative (e.g., mild, moderate, or severe) description of those symptoms that you can track from day to day. Include an updated safety assessment in every note. Make as specific a diagnosis as the data allow; update it as your understanding of the case evolves. In a sentence or two, explain your impressions of the progress of the case and rationale for your plans going forward.

Essential Personnel

As you settle into your role on the inpatient service, consider your specific responsibilities in the context of a team of professionals, each filling a critical niche in a therapeutic operation. The more you know about their roles, the more appreciative you will be for their work and the better able to coordinate your efforts.

Psychiatrist

Your role on the treatment team is to give direction and organization to the care provided to your patients. Although few, if any, of the staff work for you, they all depend on you to define the problem, diagnosis, and treatment plan that guide their work. Keep them in mind as you write your notes. Communicate with them directly in formal and informal settings.

Nurses

Hospitals are fundamentally nursing facilities, and you serve the secondary role of giving direction but do relatively little of the actual work with patients. Nurses spend hours every day interacting with patients you will see for just a few minutes. They make far more observations of specific reactions and patterns of behavior than are apparent during a brief, structured interview. They make innumerable treatment decisions within the broad parameters set by doctors' orders every day. Their understanding of and attitude toward patients set the critical tone of the therapeutic milieu in which the patient experiences a hospital stay.

To maximize their effectiveness on the front lines of care and as members of a team, take the time to learn and appreciate what they do. Explain not just your orders but also their rationale. Create an atmosphere of open and frank communication. Listen to their concerns and suggestions. Your patients will benefit from the results, and your life will be far easier.

Social Workers

Schools of social work take as foundational principles the effects on individuals and families of their interactions with one another and with the larger society, particularly as represented by government agencies and programs. This perspective greatly complements and enriches the neurobiological, behavioral, and psychodynamic approaches emphasized in medical schools.

On a practical level, their work on the treatment team most often involves communication with families, identification of community resources, and coordination of care with outside care providers. You will come to depend on these essential functions as you pursue a course of treatment. In addition, you would do well to consider their social formulation of cases, which will clarify and enrich your understanding of patients' ability to function within their family and social roles, how these contribute to their stresses, and how they will serve as resources for their recovery.

Activity Therapists

Activity therapy includes occupational, recreational, art, music, and other therapies. They have in common the involvement of physical, cognitive, and social activities, sometimes obviously therapeutic and sometimes more subtle in their benefits. Activity therapists will occasionally look to you for guidance but more often will function with a high level of independence. Make sure they have the opportunity to contribute to team meetings. Pay close attention to their observations and assessments. They will provide crucial insights into your patients' readiness to face the challenges of independent living and the nature of the obstacles that prevent it.

Patient Care Workers

With limited educational background, carefully circumscribed duties, and frequent changes in assignment, patient care workers may be overlooked as team members or interprofessional colleagues. Interestingly, among all inpatient staff, these are the most likely to turn up in a few years as your medical students, residents, and colleagues. Many are engaging in health care for the first time and are paying close attention to your attitude and interactions with patients. Even for those not on an ambitious academic trajectory, your interactions with them may have a significant effect on the quality of their work and job satisfaction.

Essential Facilities

Inpatient units vary considerably in design and patient population. Their efficiency, effectiveness, and overall environment are as strongly affected by their design as they are by policies and personnel. Make sure that the setting where you choose to work is appropriate and conducive to the type of patients you want to see and the practice you want to conduct.

Locked and Unlocked Units

Perhaps the most fundamental difference between inpatient units is whether they offer treatment on an involuntary basis. A locked unit has the option of physically preventing patients from leaving the facility because of confusion or a conscious choice to terminate care and leave against medical advice. The availability of a locked psychiatric facility is critical to ensure the safe and effective treatment of a significant subset of patients who have been deemed a threat to themselves or others or are unable to provide food, clothing, or shelter because of legally defined mental illness. The patients you will see on these units include a broad range of diagnoses and levels of acuity, making for a varied and challenging experience.

Unlocked units, by contrast, are suitable for a narrower range of patients who are willing to seek help and are more likely to engage actively in treatment throughout their stay. Your practice in this environment will be less demanding but will provide you with more opportunities to connect and develop an effective therapeutic alliance with your patients.

Involuntary Patients

Involuntary patients require a careful balance of enticement and coercion, internal and external motivation, paternalism, and beneficence. Once past the initial, often angry response to involuntary admission, many acknowledge the legitimacy and potential benefits of hospitalization. Others, because of poor insight, psychotic processes, intense emotionality, or simply an alternative vision of their lives' priorities and goals, remain opposed to psychiatric care and uncooperative with treatment. It is imperative that you consider carefully your ethical priorities as you undertake this work, maintain a level of humility and openness to consider alternative views, but feel confident in your actions with this population. For a detailed review of involuntary treatment, see Chapter 14, "Legal and Ethical Issues."

Voluntary Patients

Voluntary patients likewise cover a range of cooperation, from those who are highly motivated to be in the hospital but not to engage in treatment to those who take advantage of all that your facility has to offer. Critical tasks as you work with this group of patients include rapidly establishing a therapeutic alliance, clarifying the patient's goals and motivations, and aligning those goals with available services and realistic expectations.

Room Layout and Features

Inpatient facilities range in design from those hastily constructed in hospital space originally intended for medical patients to those carefully created with specific treatment goals in mind.

Essential features (often because they are legally mandated) include appropriate living accommodations, access to community areas, private interview space, and an immediately accessible nursing station. Safe patient rooms include both structural elements and protections against potentially dangerous patients. Little can be achieved during hospitalization if a patient feels unsafe, either from his or her own impulses or from an inpatient peer. For more on environmental issues, see Chapter 16, "Patient Safety."

Community areas are a critical component of inpatient care. The concept of a "therapeutic community" arose in the 1940s, predating the advent of effective medications for most psychiatric disorders and continuing as an important concept on modern units, albeit without many of the specific procedures recommended in early writings. Areas designated for formal and informal group activities facilitate a community atmosphere, encourage peer support, and stimulate engagement in the milieu rather than isolation and passivity.

Private interview space, either in patients' rooms or elsewhere on the unit, is critical for meaningful interaction with your patients. Honor your patients' dignity and right to privacy by using this space rather than opportunistically catching patients in hallways, dining areas, or community space. Sit down when meeting to convey your full attention and establish an appropriate atmosphere. Minimize distractions such as telephone calls, nursing procedures, and outside noises.

Interview and Activity Space

Good interviews are dependent on both solid clinical skills and a conducive environment. In general, designated meeting rooms have advantages over patient rooms for clinical interviews, primarily in their increased privacy and reduced interruptions by other staff making safety checks, taking vital signs, or recruiting patients for groups. Rooms set aside specifically for interviews have the additional advantage of not being commandeered mid-interview for a scheduled group or activity. The ideal interview room is large enough that neither of you feels crowded or uncomfortable. Chairs are neatly arranged at an appropriate distance from each other. The room is quiet and free from outside distractions. A large window facing a well-trafficked area will ensure that you are observed without any intrusion on your privacy. Exits are readily accessible to all parties. Although the multiplicity of demands on your time and the patient's may not always allow it, use these spaces whenever possible.

High-Security Areas

Although some large hospital systems, particularly affiliated with universities or other research institutes, quietly maintain "VIP" units or subunits for higher-functioning and less acute patients, a more beneficial and effective use of resources is to increase services at the other end of the acuity spectrum. A specially designated area with high staffing levels, physically separated from the rest of the inpatient unit, will provide you with an appropriate venue for the care of highly disturbed patients who would otherwise be disruptive and unsafe in the general patient community. To qualify as part of the inpatient unit and not a seclusion room, these units require a separate nursing station, community area (even for a single patient), and access to services equivalent to those provided to other patients. Nurses, activity therapists, and patient care workers often have additional training in the care of high acuity patients, creating an environment most likely to benefit these patients. Their treatment in this setting has the added benefit of preserving the tranquility and focus of the general patient community.

KEY POINTS

- Inpatient units are useful not only to maintain patients' safety but also to provide a high level of services to a range of patients who could not adequately be served outside the hospital.

- The first steps in a therapeutic process are to clarify the patient's presenting problem(s) and establish a primary diagnosis.

- Both pharmacological and psychosocial treatments are essential, but both can only be initiated, not fully experienced, during an acute hospitalization.

- Maximize the utility of documentation by writing clear, information-rich notes focused on the needs of the expected readers.

- Know and use the expertise of all members of your treatment team.

- The physical space of a well-designed inpatient unit contributes to its safety and effectiveness in creating a therapeutic environment.

- A separate high-security area benefits both the patients who require that level of care and those in the general milieu, who will be able to focus on their own treatment with minimal distraction or disturbance.

CHAPTER 3

Consultation-Liaison Psychiatry

Sarah Mohiuddin, M.D.
Wael Shamsedeen, M.D.

Consultation between medical center services—the sharing of expertise among specialists for the benefit of patients with multiple medical issues—is a well-established component of hospital-based care, but only psychiatry includes the concept of *liaison* or raises this work to the level of an accredited subspecialty. Consultation is the sharing of a medical opinion; liaison involves the offering of perspective, education of the primary team, and assistance with the unique legal, ethical, and practical considerations of mental health care.

Your work as a consultation-liaison (C-L) psychiatrist requires a unique set of skills. In addition to your psychiatric knowledge, understanding of general medical conditions, and ability to work in a high-acuity setting, you will interface with multiple services with competing demands. Many of these center directly on the best care for the patient, but some are to reduce distress within the primary team, to expedite a discharge, or to facilitate transfer to another unit.

It is easy to simplify this under the rubric of "getting the consult question right," but the "right question" may involve more than just the specific query from the consulting service. Unconscious or unspoken motivations in play, unrecognized dynamics between patient and treating physicians, and important interactions among team members often factor into a psychiatric consultation request. Because of this, as a C-L psychiatrist desiring the best care possible for your patient, you must develop the skills required not only to diagnose and treat psychiatric disorders in medical patients but also to recognize and address issues that affect patient care in each of the different medical professionals involved. This chapter serves to identify and help you navigate the unique issues that arise when working on a C-L service.

Understand the System

The culture of the institution often affects the frequency and type of consultations you are asked to provide. For example, some institutions ask for consults from all medical specialties involved with a patient, regardless of whether an active issue exists. In such cases, the frequency and volume of consults might be high, but many of those consults will be of lower acuity. The critical skill in this case is to distinguish active and urgent cases from routine, nonacute matters; to allocate your time and effort appropriately; and to communicate this effectively while still leaving open the line of communication in the event of a change in the patient's condition.

Which clinical operations are entitled to use the C-L service also varies by institution. In some medical centers, consultations are limited to admitted patients only, but in others, the C-L service covers patients seen in the emergency department, infusion centers, observation units, and so forth. In institutions without psychiatric crisis or walk-in clinics, patients may be diverted to the emergency department and ultimately to the C-L service. It is important that you understand how and where consults arise to help determine what structure and support the C-L operation may require.

The team members of the psychiatry C-L service will vary depending on the type of institution. In larger hospitals, team members may include mid-level providers, social workers, or psychologists, and your role would include leading a diverse team of professionals. Some institutions use a tiered approach to consultations, in which initial contacts are made by social workers or psychologists, and only the more acute or medically complex patients are seen by the psychiatrist. Establishing a workflow to incorporate multiple levels of team members is important to improve efficiency and establish appropriate supervision and oversight for all members of the team. In an academic medical center, the presence of medical students and residents adds a teaching component, and you may need to learn teaching skills specific to a busy clinical service (see Chapter 7, "Teaching and Supervision").

Develop Relationships With the Health Care Team

Consultations often require you to do more than address particular questions or issues related to the psychiatric management of a patient. You will function as a liaison in multiple ways: between the patient and the primary team, between the patient's inpatient and outpatient providers, and between psychiatry and the rest of the field of medicine. This liaison role is one of the unique aspects of C-L psychiatry in contrast to other areas of medicine and requires that you do more than answer a particular consultation question. As such, one of the most important aspects of your work is to establish relationships with members of the primary health care team.

Developing relationships with members of the team is like developing relationships in other aspects of your life. First, be present and responsive to the needs of the team. This is of particular importance when psychiatric concerns arise in medical settings because of the lack of knowledge and stigma that health care providers have about mental health symptoms and diagnoses. When mental health issues arise with patients in the hospital, medical providers often feel ill-equipped to address these concerns, even concerns that you recognize as simple, straightforward issues. Keeping this idea in mind when you are approached by medical teams is a key element in your ongoing relationship with the health care system. Second, spend time outside of a specific consultation to meet with teams that frequently use your services to better understand common issues and concerns that arise for them. This way, you will be able to understand what has worked well in the past, which consultations the team thought were not addressed particularly well, and what some of the common psychiatric concerns are in the context of particular medical issues.

Prepare Health Care Teams for Common Problems

Noncompliance

Consider how to address medication noncompliance in patients with chronic medical issues. You may be asked to meet with the patient to address this concern and understand the psychiatric underpinnings of this ongoing maladaptive behavior. However, you also may recognize the effect of issues outside the hospital, including impaired social supports, lack of appreciation for what the patient's medical regimen requires in terms of time and organization, and the patient's particular motivation around medication compliance. In your liaison role, you may be able to work with a team to take a broader view of the patient's needs after discharge.

Vignette

Dr. C was asked to assess Ms. L, a 26-year-old woman with type 1 diabetes, for depression and medication noncompliance. Ms. L had more than 20 hospitalizations in the previous 5 years for diabetic ketoacidosis, was admitted several days earlier for the same concern, and was recently transferred from the intensive care unit to a general medical floor. The team expressed frustration at her lack of adherence to her medication regimen and overall lack of engagement in her treatment despite their attempts to educate her while in the hospital.

During Dr. C's initial assessment, Ms. L acknowledged a history of noncompliance with her treatment regimen but struggled to describe the reasons for it. Further discussion with the social work team revealed significant psychosocial stressors, including insecure housing and impaired access to food. On repeat discussion, Ms. L described a history of early sexual abuse and neglect, poor school performance, and ongoing conflicts with her mother. It soon became apparent that her understanding of her disease and medications was limited and that lack of family support was playing a role in her overall noncompliance.

After a neuropsychological evaluation identified mild cognitive impairment, the team developed a simplified medication plan in which strategies for oversight and supervision were implemented. Social work staff were able to connect the family to outpatient diabetic support services, including regular check-ins and behavioral strategies to help with organization and planning around her diet and medications.

Aggression and Agitation

A common issue you will face is how to address aggression or agitation in the medical setting. Much can be done in planning and education around these concerns. This includes your assessment for delirium and psychosis, use of nonpharmacological approaches for agitation, addressing the safety needs of the medical team, use of psychotropic medications in an algorithmic way, and finally how to think about and manage the use of restraints in a medical setting. Just as in medical codes for cardiac arrest, when significant agitation or aggression arises on a hospital floor, it is important that the team is already prepared for the multiple scenarios that could occur in this context. The primary team will look to you as the lead for how to address these concerns. This is an opportunity to create algorithms or treatment protocols that teams can use when psychiatric support may not be immediately available. Such protocols enable the team to build on their own skills in initially addressing aggression or agitation, then to seek consultative support when those strategies are ineffective.

Teaching and Building Trust

Providing psychoeducation and building trust and relationships with the team in advance will help decrease unnecessary consultations and aid you in an acute situation when the team needs to act quickly and efficiently. Meeting with teams over time to identify common themes and issues and to provide them with appropriate psychoeducation will not only better meet the needs of the consulting teams but also minimize the potential for poor outcomes and decrease the dependence of teams on your service.

It is important when building these relationships to focus not only on physicians but also on other health care providers such as nurses, advanced practice providers, social workers, and care managers. Each member of the team plays an important role in the management of a patient with psychiatric concerns. Understanding the concerns from their perspectives will give you a sense of how to plan for psychoeducation. For example, the consulting team for an aggressive patient may be primarily interested in pharmacological interventions, but nursing staff may be more interested in how and when to use security officers, how to appropriately use restraints, and how to manage their own safety. Identifying these unique needs will allow you to address the concerns of each member of the team effectively.

Be present and responsive by having a clear plan for the management of consultations during the time that the C-L team is not physically in the hospital. Although some C-L jobs primarily require managing consultations on medically admitted patients, others may require you to cover additional settings such as emergency departments, observation units, infusion centers, or even psychiatric units. In the latter case, you may not always be able to be physically present when needs arise on medical units. This will especially be true overnight, weekends, holidays, and times when you have other important obligations. Have a clear plan of coverage for these times to remain responsive to the needs of the medical teams. Some systems ask that the team remain available by pager or cell phone. Other hospital systems have backup or cross-coverage plans to manage acute concerns that arise in the hospital. Know those systems and make sure you keep them fully informed about ongoing consultations or essential follow-up.

Other Mental Health Services

Build relationships with psychiatric services in other settings, including local inpatient psychiatric units, outpatient psychiatric clinics, and mental health professionals in emergency department settings. Relationships with psychiatrists in these settings can greatly affect your day-to-day work. Often, you will face the challenge of serving as an intermediary between these levels of care, balancing the needs of the different medical teams with the needs of other psychiatrists. One common example is a request (or demand) to transfer a patient off the medical service and onto a psychiatric unit. Medical teams are under intense pressure to discharge patients quickly when their acute medical needs are met but lower-intensity nursing care is required or disposition is delayed. However, not all patients with psychiatric diagnoses require inpatient care, and the level of medical acuity that is typically managed on a psychiatric unit differs from that which is considered nonacute to a primary medical service. As such, you will often have to provide psychoeducation to the medical teams about the level of medical care that can be provided on a psychiatric unit. These conversations become even more challenging when the psychiatric units are physically colocated with medical units. These cases often involve housing difficulties or guardianship/supervision issues that complicate disposition. The psychiatry team often has more experience in this area, and that is not a legitimate basis for psychiatric admission.

Vignette

Mr. P, a 75-year-old man with dementia and disruptive behavior disorder, was admitted to a medical unit for pneumonia from an adult care home. While in the hospital for antibiotic treatment, he was noted to be aggressive intermittently. After completion of his course of acute treatment, his previous placement refused to accept him, citing his increasing medical needs. Given the lack of a clear disposition plan, the staff became increasingly frustrated with his care.

The medical team approached the C-L psychiatry team with the request to transfer Mr. P to an inpatient psychiatric unit. Psychiatric evaluation indicated that he had a history of intermittent behavioral disruption, especially in the context of his worsening respiratory status. Records from his adult care home also showed a pattern of escalating behavior leading up to his medical admission. The C-L physician spoke with the director of the group home, who described the pattern of escalating behavior and expressed concern for having adequate staff to manage the patient given this recent escalation. The consultant was able to summarize the pattern of change and demonstrate an overall improvement in the behavior as the pneumonia was treated. However, given that the plan was for the patient to continue intravenous antibiotics for 2 weeks, the adult care home refused to accept Mr. P back until the course was complete.

The psychiatric consultant convened a meeting/case conference between the medical team, hospital administrators, and group home director to come to an agreement that Mr. P would return to the group home following completion of the course of intravenous antibiotics. The consultant then met with nursing staff and bedside staff to implement a daily schedule and predictable interventions to reduce transition-related aggression. Mr. P was able to remain for the 2-week stay without further behavioral aggression and successfully returned to his adult care setting.

In addition, maintaining relationships with outpatient psychiatrists can be equally important. When patients with chronic psychiatric illness are admitted to medical units, their treatment teams may want to change or discontinue outpatient pharmacological regimens. This could be harmful to the patient, particularly for those patients with relative psychiatric stability. Speaking with the outpatient psychiatrist can be important in understanding what changes are warranted in an inpatient medical setting. This communication also may help the medical team understand which concerns are acute or chronic, develop plans for patients with a history of aggression or agitation in medical settings, or understand how better to serve patients who are readmitted to medical units for chronic medical issues or medication noncompliance. Your communication with the outpatient psychiatrist can likewise help the medical team understand the patient's personality or behavioral traits as they manifest in hospital settings.

Get the Question Right

Getting the question right is one of the main foci of a C-L service, ensuring that the team is able to meet the needs of both the patient and the medical service. This is more challenging than it seems. Despite assertions of their importance by medical schools, psychiatric disorders and treatments remain mysterious and often frightening to other medical specialists. The medical team may intuit that something is wrong but lack the vocabulary to describe it or the conceptual framework to understand it. They may have preconceived notions about particular psychiatric illnesses, what symptoms they present with, and the time course of their treatment. Often, medical teams struggle with patients for a variety of nonpsychiatric issues, such as a communication gap, difficulty in the doctor-patient relationship, or need for intervention with a family and may seek psychiatric expertise to help address these issues. Whether these are appropriate issues for you to address remains an open question, but they illustrate an important point about how psychiatry and psychiatric issues are conceptualized by our colleagues.

"Inappropriate" consult questions are one of the most frustrating aspects of work as a C-L psychiatrist. Encourage teams to use a tiered approach to questions to help mitigate this problem. For all psychiatric services, the most pressing issues are safety concerns. From the perspective of a medical service, however, disposition of a patient whose acute medical problems have been addressed but active psychiatric issues deferred may seem equally pressing. Assist the medical team in identifying whether the consultation is about an acute psychiatric issue or is a required procedural step in preparing a stable patient for discharge. Next, establish whether the issue is a psychiatric symptom or disorder or whether the team needs psychiatric expertise to better communicate with a patient or family. Finally, clarify whether the issue needs to be resolved during the hospital stay or merely requires an outpatient referral. If you consistently address these three areas before each consultation, then it will encourage teams over time to anticipate your questions and clarify the issues involved for themselves and for you.

Ask the team to directly address certain topics before the consultation. Among these is whether the patient and family have been informed of the consultation. Often, teams will identify concerns but are reticent to share them. Encouraging the primary team to do so will not only make your job easier but also help them to engage the patient more directly in what may be a critical discussion for the patient's general medical and psychiatric care. Second, ask the team if changes have been made in psychiatric medications since admission and if it would be reasonable to resume those medications. Third, if their request involves transfer of the patient to an inpatient psychiatric unit, ask what nursing or other medical services the patient will require.

Education about psychiatric disorders ("psychoeducation") and treatment strategies for common issues like delirium and agitation will help medical and surgical teams feel competent in recognition and early management of these concerns and may decrease the unnecessary consultations. Teaching the consulting teams how to document their concerns in the chart will help the consultant understand what concerning symptoms are being noted by the team and staff and where intervention may be necessary.

It is important to highlight here that, at times, the "question" serves as a flashpoint of conflict between consultants and the primary medical team and that institutions vary widely in their cultural collegiality. The intensity of high-acuity environments can lead to stressful work interactions, particularly when they involve complex disposition issues, conflict-laden patient interactions, or stigma toward mental health conditions. It is important that interactions remain professional and respectful on all sides, and highlighting this as a priority for the C-L service will be important over time. If concerns in this area arise, try to address them first with individual teams, working to build trust and rapport and involving administration or supervisors only when other measures have failed.

Build Your Team

The Importance of a Multidisciplinary Approach

Often the demand for C-L services outstrips the ability of one physician alone to manage it. The questions or concerns raised by primary teams are as diverse and wide-ranging as acute safety concerns, untreated psychiatric symptoms, need for outpatient services, psychological or psychotherapeutic issues, and adjustment or grief reactions to medical diagnoses or traumatic events. Do not expect as a single physician to consistently do this in a meaningful way. Begin early to build a multidisciplinary team that can meet these diverse needs.

First, know your hospital and its needs. Tertiary care hospitals, with numerous intensive care beds, may have a greater volume of consultations related to delirium and withdrawal, whereas smaller community hospitals tend to be more focused on connecting individuals with depression and anxiety to mental health care after discharge. These issues should help determine the structure of your service, with more medical expertise in the first case and greater emphasis on embedded social work services on the C-L team in the second.

Second, recognize that many of these services are not reimbursable, and under the best of circumstances, C-L services are rarely self-sustaining. Be thoughtful about ways to use each staff member efficiently, maximizing the value of service he or she can perform. As a psychiatrist, focus your expertise on diagnosis at the interface of mental health and general medical conditions, pharmacotherapy, brief psychotherapeutic interventions, and education of peers and interprofessional medical teams. A psychologist can assist with cognitive assessments, behavioral plans, motivational interviewing, cognitive-behavioral interventions for insomnia and pain, and other psychotherapeutic interventions. Mid-level providers, such as physician assistants and nurse practitioners, can gather the initial history and may be able to handle routine and follow-up medication issues. A master's-level social worker can meet with patients and families, assist with placement, address outpatient resource management, and possibly do formal psychotherapy. An administrative staff member can help manage the flow of consultations by answering the initial page or call with a short series of routine questions to clarify both the needs of the primary team and the acuity of the issue. Avoid squandering these valuable resources by assigning each task according to level of training and expertise.

Build Your Skill Set

With your team in place, consider what specific skills will be most helpful for each member to develop. This will be highly dependent on the setting and types of consultations that are typically seen by the service. Under ideal circumstances, the combined skills of the team may include motivational interviewing for medication noncompliance or behavior change, cognitive-behavioral techniques for anxiety and depression, behavioral management for aggressive patients, distress tolerance skills for patients with personality disorders, medical management tools for substance intoxication and withdrawal, experience with the legal system, familiarity with insurance authorization, and understanding of documentation requirements. Educational settings require work with learners, and additional skills in teaching and education will be necessary. Ensure that each member of the team is comfortable supervising trainees in their own disciplines and is willing to share insights with other trainees.

Deal With Stigma Toward Mental Health

To a remarkable degree, stigma surrounding mental health disorders and patients is at least as prominent among health care providers as it is in the general community, perpetuated by myths that psychiatric disorders have lower validity, fewer evidence-based treatments, and less favorable outcomes than general medical conditions. Consequently, psychiatric symptoms are not recognized or addressed, medical outcomes are compromised by psychiatric comorbidities, and relationships between patients and their medical teams are impaired.

Medical personnel with limited understanding of psychiatric care tend to drift into either of two opposite fallacies: 1) that psychiatric disorders cannot be effectively treated or 2) that treatment should be immediately and completely effective (some believe both simultaneously). This may be accompanied by the well-established stigma that extends to mental health providers, including psychiatrists. Only your steady provision of prompt and attentive service, psychoeducation, and constant care in building relationships will, over time, win their confidence and begin to decrease stigma-based negative outcomes. You may also help medical teams to understand what the mental health system looks like outside of the hospital so that medical providers can learn how to better interface and navigate with outpatient psychiatrists and adjust their expectations to the strengths and limitations of local mental health services.

Address Family and Provider Conflicts

Although not properly psychiatric issues, conflicts or failures of communication between health care providers and patients or families are a frequent basis for psychiatric consultation. Rather than pushing back against these seemingly inappropriate impositions on your time and expertise, treat them as a component of your liaison function, modeling good listening skills and providing insight into the personality and stress factors that are likely hampering effective communication. As you do so, your value to the primary team and—more importantly—to the patient's welfare will be enhanced.

Anger is a common component of conflicted interactions and tends to spread quickly among all involved. Keep yourself out of the direct conflict and approach it as a liaison between the fighting parties. Make sure everyone is heard. Try to understand each position. Focus on the core issues. Identify and correct errors of fact and deficits of information. Look for common ground. Do not be too quick to label one side as wrong or unreasonable, but do not be afraid to constructively confront those problems when they are clearly present.

It sometimes becomes clear that a problem lies not with the identified patient, but with a family member (or occasionally a team member). There is no established mechanism for you to conduct a formal psychiatric evaluation on a hospital visitor, but your skills of persuasion may be sufficient. In rare cases, civil commitment procedures may even be invoked. In either case, your expertise and insights will be a valuable asset to the primary team, reducing their distress as well as the patient's and thereby improving patient care.

Conclusion

Work as a C-L psychiatrist requires a unique skill set. Work within medical settings requires you to build on your skills as a psychiatrist in terms of medical knowledge of the management of psychiatric illness and symptoms in the context of acute medical illness. However, to provide optimal care for the patient in this setting, you must also understand the needs of the medical team and address their understanding of psychiatric illness and treatment. Outcomes improve as you build a relationship with teams over time, understanding their biases and knowledge gaps and looking beyond the consult question to address stigma and fears around mental illness.

You may initially find your work in this field frustrating as each consultation requires you to intervene not only with the patient but also with the entire medical team. However, this is also what makes your work in this system immensely rewarding as the effect you have extends beyond the patient alone. You have the opportunity to teach and intervene with other medical professionals on a daily basis to increase their understanding of psychiatric illness and ultimately improve care for patients with psychiatric disorders throughout the medical system.

KEY POINTS

- Your understanding of and ability to work within the culture of your institution will affect the frequency and type of consultations you receive.

- Meet with individual services to understand what types of consultation they typically need and what psychoeducation may be useful in minimizing unnecessary consults and improving their knowledge and attitude toward psychiatric disorders.

- Medical teams should address certain issues before seeking a consultation, including safety, acuity, and whether the patient is aware of the consultation.

- In smaller hospitals, you may handle consultations alone, but in larger medical systems, it is critical to build a team of social workers, psychologists, or mid-level providers able to handle specific aspects of consultations.

- Use social work services to address disposition concerns or help patients connect to outpatient care, psychologists to address adjustment or cognitive issues, and mid-level providers to handle routine and straightforward clinical issues.

- Stigma toward patients with mental health concerns can lead to poor patient outcomes; you play a unique role in helping to address the role of stigma in the care that patients receive.

- Address stigma that medical teams have toward the field of psychiatry by building relationships over time with your fellow clinicians and staff throughout the hospital, being present and responsive to their needs.

PART II
Skill Set

CHAPTER 4

Training and Background

Gerald Scott Winder, M.D., M.Sc.

This chapter contains practical
and philosophical content that will serve both trainees and practicing clinicians contemplating a hospital-based mental health career in how to adjust
to, excel in, and enjoy the hospital environment. Although not a recognized
subspecialty, hospital psychiatry requires unique experience and expertise
that can be acquired through other specialty or subspecialty training. Several of the ideas discussed here are treated in various forms elsewhere in the
book. In this chapter, I focus on the effect of training and background experience on your success as a psychiatric hospitalist. This is not meant to
be a comprehensive review of each topic discussed, but a practical roadmap
through the types of training and background experiences that are particularly useful to psychiatrists working in the hospital.

First, I discuss the aspects of general medical education, internship and
residency, and fellowship training that an interested student or resident will
find useful in practice and should consider as part of a formative curriculum. Many of the topics discussed are sound principles for any trainee but

are deemed particularly important for those seeking a psychiatric career in the hospital environment. In the final section, I discuss features, not confined to medical training, of a clinician's general background that are useful and relevant to the practice of hospital psychiatry.

General Medical Education

As a student, medical education is not only the time when you will choose which medical discipline to pursue as a career but also the epoch when you acquire the attributes of a physician. It is the first time each of us feels what it is like to care for a patient. Intuitively, the quality of these experiences and the rigor of the supervision and teaching determine in large measure your demeanor as a developing physician. The comportment of those who teach and model for you not only plays a key role in how you perceive the discipline to which the preceptor belongs but also influences where you feel most comfortable.

Equipped with curiosity and altruism, many (if not most) matriculating students are attending their programs precisely because they want to discover in which medical discipline they will channel their passions. How the faculty view and treat patients will make an indelible impression. The psychiatric hospitalist strives to consider a patient holistically from diverse vantage points: developmental, biological, psychological, environmental, and social. Early acquisition of fluency from competent faculty in how a patient can be viewed and conceptualized through each of these lenses will position you well for a career in mental health and life in the hospital. Furthermore, medical education necessitates the deconstruction and classification of patients, their physiology, and symptoms into an array of organ systems, statistics, medical disciplines, and treatment. Although essential, this can limit future conceptualizations of the people for whom you provide care.

As psychiatric hospitalists, we desire education within a culture of rigorous science, clinicians modeling sound medical technique, while also promoting holistic views of the people who seek care for their ailments. Curricula exist, such as Rachel N. Remen, M.D.'s The Healer's Art (www.rachelremen.com/learn/medical-education-work/the-healers-art; accessed November 4, 2019), to capture and preserve personal aspects of one's own commitment to medicine while infusing medical education with a humanistic approach that can nourish both you as a clinician and your future patients. This can be an effective way to preserve early optimism and idealism in the face of the acuity and pressure of hospital work that otherwise might threaten these attributes.

The facilities of the educational institution will dictate in large part your exposure to the continuum of psychiatric care. A robust student clerkship experience entails contact with emergency psychiatry, inpatient services, consultation and liaison work, and ambulatory clinics. An understanding of the stages and tiers of care is essential for the hospitalist who must consider aspects of workup and treatment that frequently span the full psychiatric care continuum and make recommendations that will carry forward to less acute domains of care delivery.

Within the hospital, clinicians encounter the most acute presentations of psychiatric illness. Severe aspects of mood, thought, and personality disorders are common. To see them without appropriate access to faculty for perspective and debriefing not only would discourage what might otherwise be a fruitful career but also could unfavorably affect you as a student. Becoming familiar with the chronicity of psychiatric illness and learning from faculty about the value of incremental care can be a beneficial way to calibrate your role in managing these chronic conditions that frequently exist in some form over the life span rather than as conditions with clear onset and cure.

Insurance coverage and the financial means of patients can be either catalysts or barriers to their journey through the medical system. Because society is still moving toward full parity in reimbursement for psychiatric care, the psychiatric hospitalist must be aware of how private and government payers intersect with available care in the hospital and community. Many psychiatric patients find themselves struggling with lower socioeconomic status, cognitive limitations, and impairment in judgment, all of which magnify these issues, heavily influencing the quantity of care available to them and their ability to access it.

As you attend lectures on the workings of local community mental health programs, homeless shelters, and correctional facilities, or see them firsthand, you will understand how much meaningful care is delivered by nonmedical personnel and get a deeper sense of what your patients experience before and after their hospital stays and how to ally yourself with these professionals to optimize their care and outcomes.

Selecting psychiatry from the menu of available specialty options can feel like a definitive and specific choice has been made, but it can be daunting then to discover the breadth of career options available within the discipline. Even the smaller sphere of hospital psychiatry has various facets when you consider the training and credentialing required, the nature of the workday, and the culture and colleagues that you encounter. Medical schools offer robust career planning resources, student interest groups, career fairs, and lunch-and-learn meetings where invited clinicians will aid you in these important decisions.

The breadth of your medical education experience allows for only an introductory treatment of scientific philosophy, statistics, and research methods. Unless you have previous exposure to these topics, what is offered in medical school may not be sufficient if you would like to pursue an academic career and contribute to the medical literature with data-driven projects. Many medical schools allow students to take a hiatus from the medical curriculum to pursue scientific training. Understandably, the rigors of medical school can dim your enthusiasm for learning and discovery—especially on topics that are not immediately relevant to your daily duties. For the psychiatric hospitalist, however, the goal of lifelong learning will be essential to deal with the complex and increasingly integrated world of hospital-based care. Psychiatric patients encountered in the hospital will very likely present with a variety of other conditions and intersect with other specialties. You must have a large knowledge base of medicine and expertise in locating and applying information from nonpsychiatric literature and colleagues.

Internship and Residency Training

Many of the ideas mentioned as a part of general medical education can be directly extrapolated to your residency training experience. Spending time delivering care in an array of psychiatric care domains and venues is essential to appreciate the nature of psychiatric illness in the hospital as compared with a general outpatient clinic. As a resident, your faculty ideally come from different backgrounds and disciplines. It is common and desirable for neurologists, psychologists, social workers, family physicians, pediatricians, and internists to play direct and key roles in your development as a psychiatric hospitalist.

Many aspects of psychiatric residency training are controlled by accreditation bodies and are not amenable to modification or personalization. However, these required rotations (such as the internal medicine and neurology rotations during internship) offer in themselves key opportunities to acquire hospital-based skill sets. Immersion into the care delivery and operation of these services allows a high-resolution view of the practice and philosophy of medicine. The care delivered is instructive in and of itself but so is the look at how patients exist in the hospital from the acute moments of presentation to the apprehension of discharge and subsequent stages of care. During these rotations, you will see firsthand the effects of illness propagated through the patient's life, mind, and family. These key insights will inform your later hospital-based work.

Many psychiatric residency programs allow for more customization of the rotation schedule during the senior years of training. These are invaluable opportunities for the budding hospital psychiatrist to return to these services with substantially more experience to once again participate in and establish some additional expertise in the mental health aspects of hospital care. In accordance with accreditation guidelines and with appropriate supervision, elective rotations in cognitive disorders, epilepsy, movement disorders, electroconvulsive therapy (ECT), emergency psychiatry, palliative care, neuropsychology, pain medicine, and substance use disorders are particularly high-yield experiences. By no means is this a comprehensive list of electives that you might find valuable, but their relevance to the practice of hospital psychiatry is unmistakable and can pay off not only in the clinical exposure obtained but also in the contacts you make and the broader view of health care delivery you discover. Some of these electives are discussed in more detail later in this chapter in the sections on fellowship training because they also may be accessed during that phase of training.

The Accreditation Council for Graduate Medical Education (ACGME) requires that psychiatric residents receive training across the continuum of care (inpatient, outpatient, community-based, emergency, consultation, and liaison), outside of psychiatry (neurology, internal medicine), and within several of the psychiatric subspecialties (addiction, geriatric, child and adolescent, forensic, emergency). The relevance and benefit of training within the psychiatric subspecialties to a career in hospital psychiatry is discussed in detail in the following section and applies to both residents and fellows, although the exposure to the learning experience obviously will be greater for the fellows seeking specialized and immersive training in the area.

As preparation for attending status, residency programs frequently offer electives in which senior residents, with supervision, occupy the role of team attending on the inpatient unit. This entails your leadership of team meetings, staffing cases with younger residents and medical students, conducting family meetings, autonomous clinical decision-making, and caring for larger numbers of patients simultaneously. This can be an enjoyable and informative way for the hospitalist-in-training to gain direct experience with a future job. It can also offer early insight to strengths that can be leveraged and deficits that must be addressed during residency. If your training has made you aware of potential gaps in expertise or technique, you can be prepared on day 1 with a plan to address these vulnerabilities through a combination of continuing medical education, peer consultation, and supervision.

Accredited Fellowship Training in Psychiatry

Several options for fellowship training are available as you graduate from psychiatry residency. We focus initially on those fellowships in psychiatry that are accredited by the ACGME and particularly their relevant aspects to hospital practice. Following discussion of each of these training possibilities, we include some other nonaccredited training considerations of use to the hospital psychiatrist.

The discussion of each of these subspecialties is meant to highlight factors of the training that are functional and attractive to the hospital psychiatrist. The discussion is meant to convey the usefulness of exposure to this clinical work whether it exists as a shadowing and observational capacity (medical student), a limited rotation experience (intern, resident), or a designated training program (fellow). When you have undergone fellowship training in one or more of these areas, you should expect proportional levels of autonomy in conducting the clinical work within the discipline. If your exposure to the subspecialty was more limited and indirect, we would expect your expertise to lend itself more to initial detection, early phases of workup, thoughtful consultation with colleagues, and competent implementation and follow-up as appropriate within your scope of practice.

Child and Adolescent Psychiatry

To become a pediatric psychiatric hospitalist, the child and adolescent rotation is essential from all training, licensure, and credentialing perspectives. This fellowship places you in pediatric inpatient, consultation, outpatient, and emergency environments with the sole goal of future practice in one or all of these venues. You will gain essential expertise in the basic skills of inpatient psychopharmacological and psychotherapeutic treatment of pediatric patients admitted to medical, surgical, and psychiatric services. In the emergency department, you will develop expertise in gauging whether patients require hospitalization and how to navigate the effect of inpatient care on the child's symptoms, attachment, schoolwork, and family life.

Furthermore, you will begin to understand how children and their families experience treatment of illness within the medical and psychiatric units within the hospital. Evaluation and intervention on the family level are perhaps some of the most potent skill sets that the pediatric psychiatric hospitalist obtains. You will acquire a unique developmental perspective that will inform your ability to assess patients' progress along this trajectory but also allows you to be a consultant to the pediatric caregivers in tailoring other medical treatments to the children for whom you provide care.

When pediatric hospital psychiatrists are asked to assess cases of potential abuse, their training in family systems, sensitive interviewing, and establishment of a doctor-child alliance will be of particular importance. Your work in the pediatric hospital will help you appreciate the vulnerabilities of this unique population. In states where children have access to ECT, this fellowship can be a place to acquire skill in evaluating for and administering this treatment.

Geriatric Psychiatry

The advent and benefits of modern medicine guarantee that hospital psychiatrists will interact with elderly patients in each of the care domains discussed in this chapter. Expertise in geriatric psychiatry is essential to provide high-quality care to this unique patient population. As a group, elderly patients experience a greater burden of disease and concomitant medications. This creates complexity in the presentation of psychiatric symptoms and how they can be managed. Polypharmacy is prevalent, and thoughtful recommendations in this regard are an important duty of the hospital psychiatrist. Management of unavoidable drug-drug interactions is another key skill set within this training. Natural changes in different organ systems affect how medication effects are experienced, how they are metabolized and cleared from the body, and how they circulate and take effect.

Age-related conditions such as neurocognitive disorders are another high-yield component of this training. The phenotypes of these disorders are frequently behavioral, and geriatricians excel in their ability to assist patients and their families to adjust to deficits or new symptoms that appear. Geriatric evaluations are a way to hone one's appreciation of the mental status examination because this patient population shows a wide range of variability on each of the domains assessed.

When psychiatric symptoms in the elderly rise to acute levels in the hospital, geriatric training assists the psychiatrist in recommending an array of interventions and environmental modification, not just pharmacotherapy that can be overused in patients and can result in unfavorable secondary effects. Familiarity with the array of services available to the elderly (i.e., chronic care facilities, rehabilitation services, home care, and community outreach) is a beneficial perspective to have during the hospital care of an elderly psychiatric patient and planning for future phases of care.

The bedside manner of a young geriatric-trained psychiatrist can bridge the age gap and can allow elderly patients to relate to and have confidence in their youthful providers. Geriatric training provides natural interface with internal medicine, neurology, and palliative care, which themselves, as documented elsewhere in this chapter, further contribute to the development of the psychiatric hospitalist. The geriatric perspective enhances the view of the hospital psychiatrist just as the developmental perspective procured during pediatric training enriches one's view of patients and families traversing illness in the hospital.

Consultation-Liaison Psychiatry

The consultation-liaison (C-L) fellowship experience aims to equip you with the skills to evaluate and treat psychiatric symptoms in the medically ill. Inherent in the curriculum is the requirement that you become familiar with a range of medical, surgical, obstetrical/gynecological, and neurological patients. As a psychiatric hospitalist desiring expertise as a consultant and/or emergency psychiatrist, this training experience may be the most direct route to encountering the broadest sample of hospital services and personnel, medical and surgical pathology, and diverse patient populations and presentations. Although not a comprehensive list, common areas of clinical specialty and research activity that hospital psychiatrists occupy include oncology, organ transplantation, neuropsychiatry, emergency psychiatry, collaborative care, HIV psychiatry, and women's health.

The C-L experience yields a unique blend of medical and psychiatric knowledge that, if nourished and maintained, can create a sort of "amphibian" role for the psychiatric hospitalist in which he or she can comfortably inhabit multiple spheres of hospital life. This kind of training and certification has several notable benefits. From a professional standpoint, this unique blend of medical-psychiatric knowledge and expertise yields significant benefits within the hospital environment in terms of patient care, job satisfaction, and scholarly opportunities. Given the attractive features and growing popularity of collaborative care (in which psychiatry is embedded in other medical and surgical services), psychiatric hospitalists with affiliation to a particular patient population or inpatient unit find themselves in a unique and favorable position. For academic physicians in particular, the connection to a discrete segment of the hospital population is the kind of specialization that facilitates research inquiry, publication productivity, educational opportunities, and eventual promotion.

The trust developed between the psychiatric hospitalist and colleagues on a particular hospital service (e.g., transplant center, intensive care unit, cancer center) mediates several unique opportunities that you should consider. The liaison role inherent in this training allows you to understand and intervene on unique levels between patients and their medical and surgical teams. This can occur directly and on a case-by-case basis as well as more generally by improving the culture of the unit staff in terms of how they understand and approach psychiatric issues. Psychiatrists can be helpful in educating and monitoring cognitive and behavioral aspects of medical treatments (e.g., treatment adherence, lifestyle changes) that are meaningfully connected to the care the hospital unit is providing. As the unit staff trust their psychiatric consultants, they will grow more adept in their own understanding of psychiatric issues, and the quality and specificity of consultation questions will improve. This can lead to your taking an active and meaningful role in treatment planning by providing psychological and behavioral nuance to how the treatment plan is designed and implemented. Serially examining a patient population being treated by a particular service will provide unique insights into the psychiatric effects of the medications and other interventions used. As you gain credibility and trust in this role, this ability to favorably influence the care of psychiatric patients outside the mental health silo only grows.

Another unique skill set of the C-L–trained psychiatric hospitalist will be to garner understanding about how other physicians conceptualize and approach patients and how to package psychiatric information for more meaningful use, whether written or spoken. Connection to nonpsychiatric physicians throughout the hospital can secondarily lead to unique opportunities for you to influence institution policy, serve on committees, and access clinical and research resources that would otherwise be unknown or unavailable for use. Your example in working at the elbow of nonpsychiatrists also pays dividends in terms of how psychiatrists carry out their jobs, strengthening their fundamental base as physicians. Many times, psychiatrists take care of patients whose pathology is, in essence, a diagnosis of exclusion. Your experience as a hospital psychiatrist who works closely with services that perform the initial workups will solidify your understanding of the conditions that you are treating but will also help make contributions to the diagnostic picture if something has been missed or needs to be corrected. There is an ever-increasing need to identify and intervene in the behavioral etiologies behind numerous chronic diseases (e.g., liver disease, diabetes, cardiovascular disease), and the degree to which you understand their physiology, presentation, and treatment will increase your efficacy as provider and consultant. Furthermore, as increasing knowledge accumulates about biological contributors to major depression, for example, the medical expertise gained in the C-L fellowship becomes evident.

Finally, given the role of the psychiatric consultant throughout the hospital, C-L offers unique exposure to the concept of capacity to make medical decisions. This topic, widely misunderstood outside of mental health circles, is a critical area of expertise for you to develop and use not only to conduct assessments but also to teach critical principles of competency in psychiatric patients to your medical and surgical peers. This topic is covered in detail in Chapter 14, "Legal and Ethical Issues."

Forensic Psychiatry

Legal issues are a routine consideration in hospital mental health. On the inpatient psychiatry units, commitment hearings are perhaps the most direct way that hospital psychiatry intersects with the law. Forensic training focuses on, among other issues, the legal regulation of the practice of psychiatry and can provide you with unique expertise in the legal obligations of psychiatrists and the rights of patients seeking psychiatric care. For pediatric psychiatric hospitalists, competency in child abuse and neglect can be especially useful.

On the medical services, any behavior that physicians deem concerning or harmful or that directly affects safety of staff and the delivery of medical care may easily be construed as psychiatric in etiology. Forensically trained hospital psychiatrists are well positioned to comment on the hazy border between mental illness and criminal behavior. Matters of guardianship, capacity to consent, and disability, all inherent to forensic psychiatry training, are also commonly dealt with throughout the hospital. More concretely, your training in writing forensic reports can be vital when you are asked to write a letter to the courts regarding guardianship, custody, or disability.

In the emergency department, incarcerated patients present with some frequency. Forensic training equips you with an appreciation of traits of this vulnerable population and gives you additional insight into how their psychiatric symptoms present and how treatment can be implemented given their incarceration. Outside of the corrections population per se, the presence of law enforcement in the emergency department is routine given their role in responding to acute events that frequently involve mental health disorders. Forensic training will augment your collaboration with officers in properly understanding and intervening in emergent matters of behavioral health.

Hospital-based psychiatrists are frequently called on to serve as expert witnesses, both because of the high acuity of the patients seen in the emergency department and on inpatient units and because of the depth of expertise developed in dealing with these patients in the hospital setting. The core competencies of this fellowship dealing with legal statutes and the workings of a courtroom will be invaluable to you in this role.

Addiction Psychiatry

Training in substance use disorders (SUDs) will benefit you as a hospital psychiatrist in many ways. As a consultant and emergency physician, the acute phases of intoxication and withdrawal are frequently on your differential diagnosis to explain a patient's presentation. Substance use often is associated with new or worsening psychiatric symptoms, so a working understanding of the pharmacology of drugs of abuse, their intoxication and withdrawal profiles, and patterns of consumption is essential as you decide how to proceed with subsequent treatment. SUDs are highly stigmatized, and various services in the hospital can be particularly susceptible to (and unaware of) this bias. In the medical emergency department, physicians may become overly permissive in their prescribing of controlled substances out of helplessness, cynicism, and a desire to discharge the patient. Or, they may be moralistic and refuse to treat an addicted patient even when it is indicated. Organ transplant teams may allow stigma to affect a patient's access to the precious resource of donor organs, which can be lifesaving and life-prolonging. Your affiliation with these services can effect positive change in their understanding and clinical practices. Your nonpsychiatric hospital colleagues may also lack holistic appreciation for the predisposing, provoking, and perpetuating aspects of SUDs, which you can remedy by your knowledgeable interactions and trusted relationships with medical and surgical colleagues.

Many patients are admitted to inpatient psychiatry in the context of some level of substance use. At times, this requires you to actively detoxify the patient as part of the treatment plan (or detect when the detoxification requires medical consultation and/or needs to take place on a medical service). For patients whose substance use patterns are a focus for psychiatric treatment planning, the inpatient environment can be a unique venue (given the proximity of primary and secondary effects of SUD) to engage the patient psychotherapeutically. The core competencies of addiction psychiatry include motivational enhancement therapy, a paradigm and skill set that are useful for SUDs as well as for many other compulsive behaviors and lifestyle changes that inpatients may require in other contexts.

Detoxification and psychiatric stabilization are only the first phases in SUD treatment, so your familiarity with the disease course (including the stages of change and relapse) and tiers of care is highly desirable for effective treatment planning. The expertise that you gain as an addiction psychiatrist with specialized medical treatments for SUDs (e.g., methadone, buprenorphine, naltrexone, acamprosate) can be particularly valuable in hospital work because some of their utility is predicated on use proximal to or during periods of abuse. Depending on the size of the institution, access to providers comfortable with these treatments can be low, so you may find that this skill set is particularly functional.

Accredited Fellowship Training in Related Fields

Brain Injury Medicine

Brain injuries are a frequent reason for or contributor to inpatient psychiatric admissions. Although many, if not most, hospital inpatients intersect with multiple disciplines and services, brain injury patients are a prominent group within any hospital whose pathology does not fit squarely within a particular medical discipline. Indeed, injury to the brain frequently ensures that a patient will encounter numerous specialists who view the symptoms through different lenses based on training, specialty, personal philosophy, and the nature of the practice (i.e., intensivist vs. outpatient rehabilitation). Moreover, the reasons that they come to the attention of the hospital psychiatrist typically include severe and acute symptoms. This combination of factors can predispose brain injury patients to generating multiple consultations and treatment plans with numerous recommendations that may diverge or contradict one another. Training that facilitates your synthesis and practical implementation of recommendations that routinely come from numerous sources (e.g., neurosurgery, neurology, physical medicine, psychiatry, psychology, sleep medicine) is a powerful skill. Specialty training in brain injuries equips you with unique skills in assessing the myriad aspects of the condition and how they are managed. Key domains in which intensive brain injury training will benefit you include cognitive impairment; behavioral symptoms; chronic pain; autonomic, motor, and sensory deficits; and functional limitations.

Psychologists affiliated with physical medicine practices are valuable resources for hospital psychiatrists to learn ways to assist patients in accepting unpleasant symptoms or deficits and striving to maximize functioning in spite of their permanency. Brain injury medicine is a rich area for gaining insight into how multidisciplinary teams create multimodal treatment plans, stage their implementation over time, and assess incremental improvement.

Hospice and Palliative Medicine

Patients at imminent risk for death are rarely, if ever, located on an inpatient psychiatric unit for a variety of sound reasons. However, as a psychiatric consultant, you will routinely evaluate the mental health and status of persons who are struggling with a chronic medical condition. Indeed, many mental health concerns prompting inpatient consultation have direct links to concurrent disease processes, prospect of life changes, and the specter of disability and death. Accordingly, palliative care is an important, but often overlooked, node of multidisciplinary care in which you can be particularly useful.

Palliative care training requires you to acquire several unique interpersonal skill sets useful in the hospital environment. Critically ill and dying patients commonly make important treatment decisions while experiencing significant physical and psychological distress. Amidst these physiological and emotional changes, palliative physicians endeavor to limit suffering and help these patients to identify their wishes. When patients are not able to participate directly in decision-making, palliative care involves their family members in the process. This necessitates your expertise in advance directives, conflict resolution, implementing multidisciplinary and symptom-driven care, and providing meaningful counseling to bereaved individuals with an eye toward additional psychological services if needed. The attitude of caring required to excel in this type of practice is unique and is a desirable trait for a hospital psychiatrist.

Sleep Medicine

Sleep may well be to mental health what nutrition is to general medicine. Although not a perfect metaphor, it illustrates the profound effect that sleep has on the field of psychiatry. Your understanding of the fundamentals of sleep physiology, evaluation, workup, and treatment will be advantageous for inpatient mental health. You will routinely encounter patients who are experiencing insomnia as a result of medical disease; the round-the-clock rigors of hospitalization; substance abuse, active mood, anxiety, or thought disorder symptoms; and an array of primary sleep disorders. You will frequently discuss with patients and colleagues the features of their sleep elicited by clinical history, polysomnogram, and reported behaviors. Sleep hygiene and other practical recommendations surrounding sleep behaviors are routinely recommended by psychiatrists. You may order a polysomnogram as a part of a patient's workup and treatment. Many of the medications you prescribe directly affect sleep function and behaviors, favorably and otherwise. The greater your expertise in this area, the more effectively you will address these issues.

Other Useful Training Opportunities

None of the following treatments have an accredited fellowship associated with them; however, psychiatric departments routinely employ physicians and other professionals who specialize in their use. Again, the attributes that are relevant to your hospital-based psychiatric duties are emphasized.

Eating Disorders

Patients with any of the eating disorders frequently present to the hospital and require medical stabilization before psychiatric intervention. Although psychiatric in nature, eating disorders are not routinely treated on general psychiatry units. A rotation with pediatric or adult eating disorder specialists can offer insight into the acute medical diagnosis and treatment, thresholds for transfer from medicine to psychiatry, and ensuing psychiatric monitoring and interventions. Because this is another patient population that vexes medical and psychiatric colleagues alike, a broad and multidisciplinary knowledge base about the disorders can improve patient care and staff understanding of these debilitating conditions.

Electroconvulsive Therapy

ECT is a highly effective, yet highly stigmatized, procedure. Many nonpsychiatrist physicians in the hospital are not even aware that it is being done in their facility. When they find out that it is, they might relate their surprise that "we are still doing this to patients." Whether attending on the inpatient unit or consulting to the floors or emergency department, your skill evaluating for and administering ECT will be much sought after. Sometimes, patients on medical services undergoing extensive and inconclusive workups (e.g., for catatonia) or experiencing severe medication side effects (e.g., neuroleptic malignant syndrome) can benefit immensely from ECT. The hospital psychiatrist who is ECT-trained is poised to bring about these favorable outcomes.

Psychotherapy

Psychotherapy can be useful to hospital patients in myriad ways: helping them to manage their emotions and problems; giving them new awareness of what they think and feel; teaching them new ways to understand and respond to their illness, manage habits, and manage compulsive behaviors; and improving their relationships with loved ones and medical providers. These interventions range from the concrete to the abstract and can be designed to avert crisis or enhance quality of life. They can be deployed formally as, for example, groups discussing coping skills during a prolonged stay on an inpatient psychiatry unit or in a supportive context at a single patient's bedside on a surgical floor during a brief admission. Your training in how to understand grief and bereavement is also useful given their common appearance in the hospital.

Understanding the theory and practice of psychotherapy not only will enable you to use various techniques in a patient's care but also will allow for more personalized and specific recommendations for subsequent treatment plans. Psychiatric residency training and fellowship provide you with substantive opportunities to learn and use various types of psychotherapy. You may also find training and certification in specific modalities to be useful in the hospital setting.

Neuropsychology

You will often be called on to assess the cognitive status of your patients and how that affects their ability to make medical decisions or otherwise participate in their treatment course. Your ability to conceptualize the potential etiologies and presentations of various cognitive disorders is an important skill (described in more detail in the "Geriatric Psychiatry" subsection earlier in this chapter). A complementary skill is to be able to participate in the workup process in which neuropsychological testing and neuroimaging are used. Your neuropsychological colleagues (and those hospital psychiatrists with specialty training) will independently administer the tests, interpret them, and synthesize the results. However, with exposure to the neuropsychological environment, you can gain a working understanding of 1) the test structure and content; 2) the clinical indications for which they are useful, allowing for thoughtful consultation; and 3) how the information provided in the clinical report can be applied to the patients you serve.

Other Useful Background and Experience

Personal Relationships

As hospital psychiatrists, we are interested in a comprehensive view of our patients' health but also how they generally experience and react to the hospital environment. As assertive and active contributors to inpatient care, we also derive significant satisfaction from contributing positively to the broader hospital environment in which we work. We know that the hospital environment itself along with doctor-patient relationships are direct contributors to the clinical cases we are called on to evaluate. This holistic awareness includes paying attention to how the hospital and its nonpsychiatric staff address important issues surrounding mental health and substance use. One useful way that these dynamics can be more thoroughly understood and addressed is via the organic formation and maintenance of personal relationships with nonpsychiatrist physicians and other providers dispersed on various services and in unique parts of the hospital system. If pursued in a genuine way, it can provide you with personal and professional satisfaction in a durable and substantial way.

If you function in an embedded or consultation role within the hospital, personal relationships catalyze thoughtful interdisciplinary collaboration and streamline the care patients receive from their providers. Said another way, patients whose providers are closely aligned, and hold mutual trust, experience their multidisciplinary care in a more unified and cohesive way. As you collaborate with nonpsychiatrists and they get a sense of how you practice and what you are focusing on with the patient, the documentation from medical visits begins to contain additional fragments of mental health information that only improve your understanding of the patients you share over time.

The medical discipline is easily and frequently broken into arbitrary factions and tribes based on organ systems, training programs, type or phase of care delivered, professional degree(s) held, and department. Although many of these divisions are sensible, logical, and serve a purpose, they can have unfavorable side effects. Colleagues of different disciplines may come to view one another as adversaries because of clinical care issues on the floor, disagreements in treatment protocols or philosophies, or competition for limited clinical or research resources. Reputations of individual clinicians or the services on which they attend may be propagated and become ingrained in the culture. Many of these entanglements can be averted by personal relationships and meaningful collaboration. Fruitful secondary effects of developing widespread personal relationships within a hospital include invitations to sit on committees, professional networking, and access to clinical and research resources that would otherwise remain undetected to the more isolated hospital psychiatrist.

With the busy pace of hospital life, worthwhile relationships with nonpsychiatrists are more likely to form when they are sought out and maintained. There is little reason to suppose that these relationships will develop automatically. In academic centers, services are staffed by residents and fellows, which removes the usual conversations between attendings, whose appointments in the hospital will outlast those of their trainees. Faculty research efforts may further sequester us away into niches of our respective expertise and away from the common areas of hospital life. Worse, whole bodies of personnel belonging to different departments may grow at odds based on care-related issues, tradition, or any number of political reasons. In short, the more that modern medicine becomes hyperspecialized, and in the absence of interdisciplinary affiliation, our ways of thinking about medical problems and relating to one another can become limited and stagnant. This may decrease your level of collaboration and secondarily affect meaningful patient and system-based outcomes.

Associating personally with providers outside of your discipline allows an up-close and candid view of how they encounter and conceptualize patients cared for on their services. It helps you see the value in and learn from other medical disciplines, training backgrounds, and treatment philosophies. As a psychiatrist, you should value a fresh look at yourself and your profession from a different angle. This rich information broadens your own views about what contributes to patient experiences throughout our health system and enlightens you as to why and how mental health issues may be more optimally addressed in one area of the health system when compared with another. Furthermore, if problems are to be identified and remedied, then an extant personal relationship and trust will catalyze the needed inter-provider discussion and education. This is a highly effective way to constructively and collaboratively combat insidious stigma that may shade patient experiences in your hospital.

Embedded Providers

Collaborative care (in which a psychiatrist is practicing in a "nonpsychiatric" environment such as a medical clinic, trauma or burn intensive care unit, or general emergency department) is an effective clinical trend in the field, and many believe it will embody a large part of how psychiatric care is delivered to the medically and surgically ill. Psychiatrists working next to medical and surgical colleagues in this format is a pathway to innovation. This is of the utmost importance to the hospital psychiatrist.

As more hospitals see the value of leveraging embedded mental health providers on medical and surgical services, increasing numbers of novel care delivery models will emerge in various specialties. As discussed in more detail earlier (see subsections "Consultation-Liaison Psychiatry" and "Personal Relationships"), the development of working personal relationships within the hospital will poise you to fill these collaborative opportunities and excel in your work. Many of these clinical opportunities come with significant research and education potential. They may range from care delivery as a primary mental health provider in tandem with medical colleagues to a more detached role in the context of provider-to-provider consultation. Downstream, medical students and other trainees will see this integration and the fundamental connections between brain, behavior, and body and develop more favorable views of psychiatric patients, providers, and practice that may color their career choices and also how they deliver clinical care as attendings.

Decisions to hire psychiatrists to these unique positions are often logically predicated on finding the right match of expertise and personality to blend well with the existing culture of the medical unit. This only magnifies the importance of the personal and professional issues already discussed in this chapter. As you develop into an assertive, competent, and approachable member of the hospital community, doors leading to novel embedded clinical models will open, and you will be equipped to excel in the care you deliver and the outcomes you strive to improve.

Continuing Medical Education

As a hospital physician, you are caring for acutely ill individuals whose symptoms frequently extend far beyond your individual scope of practice. This work requires a dynamic and working knowledge of broad medical principles as well as a practical understanding of how to navigate the medical literature when an explanation or solution eludes you. You will benefit from remaining in touch with lectures and seminars inside and outside of your discipline to both refresh what you have already learned and broaden your personal understanding of modern medical progress. You should seek out training (from medical librarians, for instance) on efficient access to the primary medical literature by using sophisticated online search platforms and databases. Attending the grand rounds of other departments when topics are of interest to you is a way to expand your medical knowledge while visibly showing an interest in physicians from other disciplines. As you negotiate or revisit the terms of your employment, this is a good time to ask for annual funds that would allow you to travel and participate in national conferences where these topics are discussed in detail by national experts. This fulfills not only your personal commitment to education but also those formal requirements by licensing and certification bodies that track your ongoing education.

As motivation toward these pursuits, you need only consider together the broad physiological effects of the medications you prescribe, the ever-expanding pharmacopoeia that hospital patients are exposed to, and the endless variability of the individual patients you care for to see the value in committing to a pattern of lifelong learning in this way. You need this level of preparation to be at your best. If you look beyond the medical aspects of your expertise to the more psychological and behavioral contributors to your patients' disorders, you appreciate the value in maintaining a working repertoire of psychotherapeutic skills. This allows you to actively intervene in whatever capacity you find yourself in but also to make thoughtful referrals to colleagues when the psychotherapeutic intervention your patient needs exceeds what you can offer in your hospital unit. Ongoing psychotherapeutic training and supervision through the university or local institute is a way to accomplish this, as is working alongside psychologists, therapists, and social workers who maintain these skill sets.

Administrative and Committee Roles

Becoming a contributing member of the hospital community will pave the way toward administrative opportunities. This solidifies and concentrates your role in effecting positive change for psychiatric patients. Facility, local, and regional practices can be shaped by thoughtful, trusted, and broad-based psychiatrists who know how their colleagues think, understand the way the hospital functions, and have the trust of those in their professional circles. As more psychiatrists occupy roles of this kind, the prestige and reputation of psychiatry can evolve and improve in ways that may yield additional opportunities big and small (see Chapter 6, "Leadership and Administration," for more on this topic).

On-Call Duties

Most, if not all, hospital psychiatrists are required to be on-call. This may include responsibilities for the patients admitted to psychiatry, speaking to colleagues at other hospitals about transfers, consulting with nonpsychiatrist colleagues about their own inpatients, or triaging and collaborating with emergency physicians. Your attitude while serving in the capacity of psychiatrist-on-call can greatly improve the quality of the experience and what you gain from it.

You can enhance your on-call experience in myriad ways. Consider a psychiatrist receiving a call from a general emergency department physician as an example to explore this idea. The hurried emergency department physician may need assistance in managing his own strong emotional reactions to a particular patient or patient group. Words of acknowledgment and empathy before diving into the details of the case may help to alleviate his frustration and be a point of education about the nature of psychiatric problems that present in this way. As a peer who can convey general medical knowledge alongside our psychological and behavioral insights, you can foster feelings of trust and good will. Your emergency colleague may provide you with a more complete and accurate depiction of the patient being evaluated, thus facilitating better recommendations from you. He may be more likely to answer your questions about the case and what medical conditions he may be considering alongside the psychiatric issues at hand. He may be more willing to answer questions you have about the case or other medical principles and procedures. Having gained his confidence, you can set reasonable expectations about the realities of treatment availability, time to effect, and potential pitfalls. Leaving the encounter, both of you will experience mutual positive sentiment.

Supervision and Mentorship

The variety in the clinical work of the hospital psychiatrist is seemingly infinite. As such, having access to colleagues for consultation, second opinions, and supervision is highly useful. This allows you to monitor your own reactions to patients and colleagues and gain insights and ideas from those who share your profession but possess their own form of practice.

The pace and intensity of hospital life can become a burden at any time during the arc of your career. Physicians carry several mental health risk factors by the nature of who we are and the jobs we do. Surrounding yourself with trusted colleagues inside and outside the department of psychiatry can help you balance work and personal matters as well as make decisions about what hospital services to include in your professional repertoire. In turn, becoming this kind of colleague to others yields its own personal and professional benefits and contributes to a wholesome hospital work environment.

Research

Many chronic diseases commonly treated in the hospital have behavioral etiologies. Others have psychological factors as perpetuating factors. The training of your colleagues may not have provided them with the expertise to address this adequately in a scholarly fashion, which creates a unique niche for the hospital psychiatrist to become an integral part of a multidisciplinary research team. As you affiliate with nonpsychiatrists in the research domain, you will discover funding sources that you might not have otherwise been aware of, which, in a time of increasing competition for research money, could mean everything to a developing project.

KEY POINTS

- Although not a recognized subspecialty, hospital psychiatry requires unique experience and expertise that can be acquired through other specialty or subspecialty training.

- Accredited fellowship training, particularly in consultation-liaison psychiatry, may provide valuable in-depth experience and open additional employment opportunities.

- Consider closely allied nonpsychiatric training, such as sleep medicine, pain medicine, or palliative care, to fill essential niches in hospital settings.

- Additional nonaccredited training may enhance your abilities in specific activities and roles, such as performing electroconvulsive therapy.

- Develop relationships with colleagues both inside and outside psychiatry for mutual advice and support.

CHAPTER 5

Career Development in the Hospital Setting

Michael D. Jibson, M.D., Ph.D.

Career development means
different things to different people in different settings. Within the clinical world of a private office, it may refer to the development of unique expertise and recognition for specific experience and skills, the creation of a treatment setting that reflects your own goals and values, or the acquisition of a group of patients whose care is particularly rewarding. In a larger, more structured setting, it may include administrative roles that require and develop leadership skills; collective vision; and oversight of others' work, careers, and professional growth. In the public sector, these factors may be augmented with leadership in county, state, or federal hierarchies that oversee and manage community mental health agencies, U.S. Department of Veterans Affairs clinics and hospitals, or services within correctional facilities. Within a university department, all of these roles may be complemented by academic ranks that reflect the recognition of peers for research, teaching, or other activities.

In this chapter, I focus on the effect of a hospital-based career on each of these issues, including the degree of flexibility in type and setting of practice, opportunities for professional growth, potential leadership roles, and the types of career recognition that may be expected. The hospital setting is uniquely circumscribed, both physically and conceptually, and the decision to focus primarily on this venue comes with a particular set of opportunities and limitations. Both the choice to set out on this career track and your satisfaction over the course of a career require a clear understanding of these issues.

Job Satisfaction

To a remarkable degree, physicians in general and psychiatrists in particular are sufficiently in demand that you should be able to choose or craft a job and a career track that reflect your unique interests, skills, and goals. In every setting, however, it quickly becomes clear that you are never free from the demands of patients, families, payers, and regulators. Even the most broad-based practice is not free of routine and repetition. It seems that even in this field, with its endless variety and opportunities, there is always the potential to feel trapped or exploited. In choosing a career path, it is critical that you fully recognize the qualities that make a job rewarding and renewing for you rather than draining and constricting.

Routines of Care

Several keys to job satisfaction are most important at the opening phase of a career. The first is to find the routine that best fits your interests. Closely related to this is to find the variety hidden in the routine that will keep your interest engaged.

Hospital-based services are characterized by high acuity and rapid turnover. Patients are likely to present to a hospital emergency department or inpatient unit with a handful of typical complaints, acute suicidality almost certainly topping the list. Most psychiatric disorders are worsened by substances, and you can expect a far higher percentage of cases to be complicated by intoxication in these settings than in most outpatient clinics. Psychosis mostly shows up in a narrow spectrum of outpatient venues but occurs with high frequency in the hospital. Delirium is rare in the community but is a mainstay of consultation-liaison services. These cases form the routine of hospital-based patient populations. They need to be a source of interest and engagement for a hospitalist career to be viable.

One of the most effective ways to do that is to find the variety within the routine. Suicidality may be ubiquitous in the emergency service, but the story leading to its presentation and the path you navigate together to guide its treatment will likely be unique. One reason check-box approaches to evaluation are so rarely effective is that they omit the stories that form the essential background, stories filled with nuance and novelty. Even when the time for assessment is short and the conversation focused, the investment of a few minutes to hear the patient's story will have a powerful effect on the patient's experience, the case's outcome, and your satisfaction.

The emotional experiences of patient, family, and friends are often novel to them even when the clinical presentation is common for you. All clinicians have the opportunity to recognize and work with the patient's experience, but as a hospital-based psychiatrist, you will have more opportunities to diagnose a first episode of illness and explain its nature and implications to a patient and family than will those seeing patients in other settings. In these moments of extreme distress, your familiarity with the environment, comfort with the clinical situation, and expertise in navigating treatment systems are intensely important to all concerned, especially those for whom this is an unknown and terrifying experience. Your comfort and skill with this routine make you effective and every encounter engaging and vital.

Competence, Proficiency, and Expertise

One great advantage of routine is the development of expertise with the problems you are most likely to encounter. Every new trainee is familiar with the transition from novice to competent practice, as the rote rules of assessment and tables of treatments are gradually committed to memory, become so familiar that they are unconsciously consulted, and are finally incorporated into a more intuitive understanding of disorders and therapies. Research on this maturation of professional skills highlights the importance of repetitive experience on the development of higher-level expertise. This by-product of routine is among its most satisfying consequences.

This is especially true in high-acuity, short-term situations, in which anxiety runs high for providers and patients alike. Ironically, for the "adrenaline junkie" drawn to the hospital setting to avoid the slow-paced patterns of outpatient care, it is comfort with crises and familiarity with available interventions that make for a successful career. Your ability to assess a situation rapidly and accurately and to intervene effectively is essential; your capacity to do so without your pulse rising is an inevitable outcome of growing experience and the emergence of pattern recognition, which constitute expertise. This expertise is the gift of routine and is one of the great satisfactions of having a job with common elements that you enjoy.

Sense of Purpose

Among the factors that make for a satisfying career is your sense of the significance of the work you do. Most communities and populations are significantly underserved for psychiatry in all forms, and the care that is provided in nearly every setting is offered in the midst of shortage, but some settings have greater needs than others. For those whose motivations in medicine include a desire to serve the underserved, hospital settings may provide an ideal medium for doing so.

Emergency department and hospital-based care by their nature are filled with crises and pivotal moments in the lives of patients and families. Individuals without adequate health care resources may first seek care in the midst of these crises. This essential safety net serves not just to catch those whose outpatient services are temporarily overwhelmed by their distress; for large segments of the population, it represents the entry point for care they might otherwise not receive.

Hospital services are not and should not become the primary source of ongoing mental health care, but they may provide access to services for which the individual may not otherwise have qualified or could not have located without assistance. It is common for patients to arrive in the emergency department without established care or an understanding of how to find that care. It is far less common for patients to leave the hospital without at least some type of follow-up. Most of this critical identification of services is provided by skilled and dedicated social workers and case managers, but the psychiatrist has the essential responsibility to define the condition to be addressed and the most appropriate treatment to provide. Your understanding of that role will make you an invaluable asset to this population and to the overall health care system.

Vignette

Dr. A had just finished residency and was eagerly beginning a fellowship before entering practice. To make ends meet, she designated a few hours each week for moonlighting in a private office, where she continued seeing several of the psychotherapy patients she had treated during residency. She enjoyed the work and appreciated the full fees, paid directly by the patients, that she received. She began to notice, however, in the waiting room, which she shared with several psychologists and social workers, that they were serving a narrow spectrum of patients and that many therapists in her upscale community were vying for the 20% of the population that could afford their services. This gnawing realization became of sufficient concern that Dr. A gradually shifted her clinical time to the public sector, first working at a community mental health clinic, then taking a position at an understaffed public hospital nearby, finding the job setting more satisfying and giving her a greater sense of purpose.

The Patient Relationship

The hospital-based psychiatrist's role is more often focused on crisis intervention than on the establishment of a long-term working relationship, but the same principles of listening, empathic understanding, and constructive support will serve your patients in this setting as well. In reality, the ability to build such a relationship is as critical here as in any outpatient clinic. The important differences are that it must be established quickly and without enhancement of dependence or implications of abandonment. With these boundaries firmly maintained, such relationships can be as important to the patient's recovery and to your satisfaction as they are in other less acute settings.

Your ability to establish rapport quickly with an acutely ill patient is a core clinical skill that is taught and assessed throughout training. It lays the foundation for communication of not only sensitive clinical information but also the subtler underpinnings of personal meaning, contextual relationships, and operative personality traits. Equally important, it facilitates the trust that is essential to engage the patient in the critical process of self-disclosure and commitment to treatment and wellness. There is some truth to the adage that the psychiatrist in the emergency department has to make only one decision—to admit or not to admit—but the ability to make that decision correctly depends to a large extent on the quality of that brief relationship and its meaning to you and your patient.

The first step in this process is to listen patiently. This may seem counterintuitive in the hospital setting, but it is as true here as elsewhere. The difference in this environment is what constitutes patience. Physicians in general, and emergency physicians in particular, are notoriously hurried in their information gathering, rarely tolerating more than a few seconds of silence or more than a sentence or two of elaboration. The investment of 5 minutes to listen to a patient's story will not upset the schedule but may make the difference between a meaningful and effective intervention and a mechanistic treatment with little benefit.

Vignette

Mr. B was a first-year medical student assigned to a busy urgent care clinic for his initial training in physical examination skills. He nervously watched as a 65-year-old woman with a history of mild congestive heart failure came in with worsening shortness of breath. Mr. B watched as the attending asked the usual questions about the duration, intensity, and frequency of the symptoms, keeping the discussion focused on her cardiovascular function despite her repeated attempts to wander off topic. Mr. B noticed, however, that she was not just rambling but kept trying to explain that she thought "it all started" when she got news that her 40-year-old son, who lived in another city, was hospitalized with chest pain. The attending was focused on helping Mr. B hear the crackles with his stethoscope that confirmed his diagnosis. Having completed the examination and written appropriate orders, the attending arranged for her admission and moved on to the next case, discussing with Mr. B the finer points of pulmonary auscultation.

Mr. B returned the following week and ran into the attending in the hallway, who stopped to give him an update. "It was the strangest thing; nothing we did improved her breathing until her son, who heard she was hospitalized, flew in. As soon as she saw that he was okay, her lungs cleared right up." Mr. B made a note that rales were not the only thing he needed to listen for when seeing a patient in an acute setting.

Work Environment

The social environment of your workplace will have a profound effect on your enjoyment of every aspect of your job. Collegiality and mutual respect among professionals will contribute as much as your schedule and patient population to your job satisfaction. Curiously, this realization has not penetrated every setting equally, and a wide range of attitudes prevails across medical systems. Seek a position where your work and expertise are valued, where you feel respected and included.

Contribute to a positive atmosphere by being a good citizen and collaborator. Participate in governance and service to the health system. Be generous with your time and knowledge. Look for opportunities to interact in positive and constructive ways. Be friendly and welcoming to newcomers. Promote the ideals of diversity, equality, and inclusion not merely in reference to specific populations but also in every interaction.

If you can do nothing else, create a positive microenvironment within your own treatment team. Be respectful of allied health professionals' training, skills, and work. Take the time to learn what they do. Observe and emulate their effective patient interactions. Respect them enough to share your thinking about cases, your areas of uncertainty, and the rationale for your treatment plans. Maintain an open mind about their perspectives and opinions. Learn to trust their judgment and abilities. When they have deficits in those areas, work with them to build appropriate skills. These are the elements of team leadership, rather than simply management, and they will go far in determining the quality of your work environment and satisfaction.

Autonomy and Control

Learned helplessness is a pattern of passivity and despair acquired by long exposure to an unpleasant situation over which you have no control. In contrast, empowerment and self-determination are associated with satisfaction and personal growth. Although these general rules are partially a function of individual personality traits, they apply at least as well in the work setting as in other aspects of life. This is particularly true for the dominant, driven, high-achieving character of many who are attracted to the demands of medical training and practice. Your job satisfaction will require a significant measure of control over your work setting, patient type, and clinical flow.

Although this may appear challenging in hospital settings, you have control over significant areas. Specifically, great differences are seen in the work done within various hospital settings. Emergency work is fundamentally different from inpatient care and bears little similarity to a consultation service. Hospitals likewise show a broad range of acuity and volume in the patients they serve. At a more detailed level, hours per day, days per week, and weeks per year can be negotiated. Consider each of these issues as you select and craft your job description.

Most important, however, is your control over the management of the care you provide. Within each setting, it is critical to take ownership of the operation of your clinical service, assignment of responsibilities to team members, and arrangement of treatment plans. One of the greatest determinants of satisfaction for clinicians is their ability to guide and direct care, even while empowering allied professionals working within their own spheres. Clinical care is most rewarding when it involves active thought and proactive planning, direct engagement in the processes of care, and attention to the nuances of each case. Be engaged at every step, and you will have no trouble finding both liberty and satisfaction in the care you provide.

Physician Well-Being and Burnout

Closely allied with job satisfaction is physician well-being, which is negatively correlated with its opposite, personal and professional burnout. Burnout is more than job dissatisfaction; it is the loss of motivation and reward that is essential to maintain a vibrant and growing career. It is reflected in haphazard work habits, flagging interest in routine tasks, and disengagement from both the goals and the processes of clinical care. It may include a growing sense of professional nihilism, with waning confidence in our ability as a field to meaningfully diagnose and treat psychiatric disorders or to genuinely effect change in the trajectory of our patients' lives. Mere data demonstrating psychiatry's effectiveness in these areas do little to address a loss of faith by a disaffected practitioner.

Sources and Consequences

Some sources of burnout are delineated in the previous paragraph. Others include an excessive workload, hostile work environment, isolation, and institutional goals at variance with personal priorities. As these negative factors accumulate, without a corresponding growth in factors that promote resilience, your risk grows.

Beyond the loss of job satisfaction and professional effectiveness, burnout carries over into your personal life, relationships, and capacity for constructive recreational activity. Although burnout is not a formal psychiatric diagnosis, it is closely associated with depression, anxiety, trauma, and substance use disorders. The development of such a pattern tends to be self-perpetuating and potentially devastating.

Recognition and Treatment

Recognition of the need for positive attention to physician well-being has grown steadily in the past decade. Excellent resources are available through the American Psychiatric Association and other professional organizations, as well as within many medical systems. Fundamentally, these programs consist of three core components: screening tools, personal support, and workplace modification.

Screening Tools

Screening tools range from narrative descriptions of the causes and consequences of burnout (such as this chapter) to formal questionnaires that score your responses and compare them with population norms. They are useful in clarifying and validating negative feelings that may not have been clearly delineated or acknowledged and serve as an objective reality check to use in deciding whether further steps are justified and appropriate. Several such tools are available online for anonymous use.

Personal Support

Personal support covers a range of relationships, including intimate partners, children, and close friends. These relationships are essential to well-being and are often the first to suffer the consequences of burnout. Pay attention to them, protect them, and involve them in your plan for personal and professional well-being. In addition, your involvement in a community or variety of communities can add greatly to your personal resilience and management of stress.

Social, professional, religious, service-based, or interest-based groups will provide you with a sense of belonging that directly counters personal and professional isolation. They bolster your sense of self and purpose in parallel with whatever identity you derive from your work. The renewal they provide will carry over into your professional life in important ways by defining the boundaries of your job commitments, providing a basis for leaving work behind both physically and mentally at the appropriate times.

Professional intervention in this regard should not be overlooked. Supportive or exploratory psychotherapy, mindfulness training, relaxation exercises, distress tolerance, and other modalities all have their place in the promotion of physician wellness. In previous generations, this was considered an essential component of psychiatric training. This context is new, but the effectiveness of the intervention is well established.

Vignette

Ms. C was an activity therapist on an inpatient team of three psychiatrists on a busy clinical and research inpatient service. Noting that several of the physicians seemed stressed, she invited them to participate in a specially scheduled activity therapy session on stress management, where she asked each of them to complete the sentence, "I know I am under stress when…." To model the kind of answers she was looking for, she explained that she knew she was stressed when her neck and shoulder muscles tensed and she began avoiding her email. The doctors looked puzzled and incredulous until one finally answered, with a touch of sarcasm, "…when I'm awake," and another followed with "…when I'm breathing." They sat through the rest of the session politely, then rushed back to work. A year later, only one of them still worked there, marveling that Ms. C had been there more than 25 years.

Vignette

Dr. D chaired a group working on the restructuring of the hospital's adult inpatient unit. A high priority was the replacement of unstructured activities with therapy groups based on cognitive-behavioral and dialectical behavior therapies. A nurse jokingly observed that identification of thought distortions, distress management, distress tolerance, and interpersonal effectiveness would help the staff as much as the patients. Less amused than intrigued, Dr. D scheduled cognitive-behavioral and dialectical behavior therapy "training" sessions for interested staff. They proved to be both popular and effective, including among the hospital-based psychiatrists.

Workplace Modification

Workplace modification is often overlooked as a legitimate option to address an unfavorable work environment. Although some issues are difficult to alter, such as payer expectations regarding documentation, other issues may be negotiable and amenable to change. Work schedules, patient loads, ancillary activities, tasks not requiring physician involvement, and similar issues may require only attention and motivation to change, often with mutual benefit to all concerned. Keys to success in doing so include your understanding of the reasons for current policies and procedures, involvement of all stakeholders, clarity about your goals in making a change, and good negotiating skills.

In the current social environment, your well-being is generally considered an appropriate basis for a request or proposal for change. This is especially true if you can cite negative consequences, including stress and burnout, as the impetus for the request. Positively framed, constructive proposals are the best received and most likely to be enacted. Your willingness to be part of a workgroup to review the issue and outline appropriate actions will further increase the probability of meaningful changes.

Vignette

Dr. E was part of a rotating team of inpatient psychiatrists on a 30-bed inpatient unit at a university hospital. For several years, each attending spent 4 months per year managing a 15-patient team, with other months distributed among other services and faculty activities, such as teaching and research. The large teams were grueling to manage, and turnover among faculty was high. Dr. E proposed that the unit be organized into 3 teams of 10 patients and that each attending staff the unit 6 months of the year. Despite the chair's initial concerns about the loss of 2 months of academic time for each faculty member, a trial period showed that turnover was reduced, and productivity remained high. Five years later, no one had left the service.

Professional Growth, Promotion, and Leadership

A fundamental difference between a career and a job is the expectation of growth and advancement. Within the hospital environment, the opportunities for both are plentiful, even if the range of services provided is fairly circumscribed.

Skill Development

Narrowly defined responsibilities and repetitive tasks may allow you to develop great skill, or they may just lead to rigidity of practice, as habits you carry from residency gradually come to be seen as "clinical wisdom." The difference between those two outcomes is mostly determined by the attitude you bring to each new encounter. Skill develops as you work to learn from each experience, looking beyond the patterns that emerge from two or three cases to more meaningful reflections after seeing dozens or hundreds, combined with consistent effort to stay connected to high-quality research studies and expert clinical guidelines. The difference between growth and stagnation is often as simple as a willingness to try something new or to make a decision based on published data rather than personal preference.

More formal skill development may involve courses at professional meetings, consultation with a visiting expert, or even a return to fellowship training. For skills that can be incorporated in routines of care, such as motivational interviewing, a workshop may be sufficient to get started, after which the skill can be honed with practice, further reading, and refreshers at future meetings. For procedures, such as provision of electroconvulsive therapy or laboratory diagnosis of sleep disorders, specific credentialing is required. Formal training is usually expected and may consist of a defined period of instruction and supervision. For entry into a broad new area, such as child psychiatry or addictions, a fellowship will provide a broader and deeper experience and knowledge base than is usually attained by the routines of patient care in practice. In each case, some effort is required to learn a new skill, after which an entirely new tool becomes available to you and your patients.

Promotion

Rank

Rank is a concept universally employed in academics and the military, involving clear expectations for each level and a formal process of advancement. Health care organizations may use similar concepts to recognize experience and unique expertise, with titles that reflect advanced standing within the organization. Medical systems have plentiful opportunities to achieve promotion within the hospital setting. Each institution defines its own criteria, but these generally follow a few standard patterns.

Within the realm of academics, entry-level faculty are typically designated as instructors or assistant professors and meet a standard of having achieved or demonstrated potential for local or regional recognition by peers for research, leadership, clinical expertise, or teaching excellence. Associate professors have attained regional or national recognition in one or more of these areas as judged by peers inside and outside the institution, and professors are attested by peers from around the nation to have achieved this at the national or international level. At each level, the critical requirement is recognition by peers and evidence of effect in an ever-widening circle. Fundamentally, academic promotion is about becoming known and respected for some type of academic endeavor, most often through publication or participation in professional organizations.

Tenure Versus Clinical Tracks

Tenure versus clinical tracks are commonly distinguished in university settings, largely based on the expectations laid out in your job description. Tenure has long been the fundamental sign of academic legitimacy, a badge of trust conferred by the institution on individuals whose acumen and productivity are considered beyond the need for continued review. Until the 1990s, nontenured clinical track faculty were generally clinicians hired to

cover patient-care services to free up tenure track faculty to teach and conduct research, the core functions of medical school faculty. Clinical track
faculty generally had no scheduled time away from clinical duties to engage
in academic activities and rarely sought or achieved promotion. Several factors led to a gradual shift in these faculty roles and the realities of their day-
to-day assignments.

The first factor was an increasingly competitive environment for research funding, leading to greater demands for investigator time and dedication to research at the expense of teaching and clinical effort. Tenure track
faculty who had previously been scheduled with equal time devoted to these
three core functions were forced to narrow their focus or lose access to
grants. Promotion was based primarily on production of peer-reviewed papers and continued grant support, whereas clinical work provided no such
rewards, and teaching was an expectation with little recognition or accountability.

Second, clinical track faculty found themselves increasingly called on as
medical educators, initially as bedside supervisors, then as classroom teachers, and ultimately as education administrators. Leadership roles followed,
first on clinical services, then in medical school administration. These roles
provided new opportunities for publication and other recognition, leading
faculty to seek promotion and standing as full-fledged rather than second-
tier faculty members. By the early 2000s, much of what was traditionally
considered academic life had been transferred to clinical track faculty,
whereas the tenure track was increasingly narrowed to research faculty
whose qualifications for promotion had less to do with how many papers
they published than with how reliably they received grant support to cover
their salaries.

Hospital-Based Activities Leading to Promotion

Hospital-based activities leading to promotion now abound for clinical
track faculty in most settings. Although a few high-intensity research universities maintain hospital units primarily to conduct research, these remain the exception and the domain of individuals whose career tracks are
focused on research rather than clinical care. For most institutions, hospital
services are designed primarily for clinical care, the defining characteristic
of the hospitalist. Within this context, academic excellence and leadership
may be demonstrated by developing a specific area of clinical expertise, providing exemplary or innovative teaching, or using your clinical cases to address specific research questions. Satisfying as these activities may be in
their own right, to be effective for promotion, they must be disseminated
through peer-reviewed publications, posters and workshops at professional

meetings, or participation in committees and work groups within and across institutions.

Publication has long been an essential function of academic life, yet writing skills are rarely taught or rewarded in medical school or residency. Good mentoring and consistent practice are key elements. Appropriate topics are best found within the routines of your work. Brief reports of interesting cases are readily apparent when you begin looking for them. Best practices with specific groups of patients with whom you have extensive experience make excellent topics for clinically informed reviews. Innovative practice patterns that you have developed, with or without outcome data, may be of interest to others struggling to find ways to provide the same care.

Vignette

Dr. F had spent 25 years working in a community hospital affiliated with a nearby medical school that sent clerkship students to rotate on his inpatient service. Always a favorite of the students, he enjoyed supervising them and had been the recipient of several teaching awards for his work. He was surprised and gratified when approached by the medical school to take over as director of the university hospital inpatient unit and to become a clinical assistant professor. Much of the work was essentially identical to what he had been doing before, with the addition of residents on his service as well as medical students. He was anxious, however, to try his hand at publishing but was unsure how to approach this. With a little encouragement from a senior faculty member, he began writing reviews about the topics he dealt with every day, such as inpatient use of medications, appropriate application of psychotherapy in acute settings, and the organization and management of an inpatient service. He soon had an impressive body of publications and was on his way to promotion.

Research topics that can be addressed without external funding or dedicated research time are similarly plentiful on hospital services. Many electronic medical records are designed to facilitate data extraction to address a variety of clinically relevant questions from existing cases. The effectiveness of specific interventions to prevent suicide, avoid falls, minimize risk of deep-vein thrombosis, reduce rebound admissions, facilitate adherence to follow-up care, motivate patients for substance use treatment, and countless other issues encountered daily in the hospital setting make ideal topics for study. For retrospective studies, approval of your institutional review board is essential but readily navigable. Find a senior faculty mentor to guide you through the initial steps, and you may be surprised by how accessible these projects are.

Teaching skills are much valued by learners and institutions alike, but they are independent of content expertise and must be developed separately. The skills required for classroom didactics, bedside teaching, or global supervision are not equivalent, and each requires a unique approach. These issues are addressed in detail in Chapter 8 ("Initial Assessment and Treatment Planning") and are mentioned here only in the context of promotion. Recognition of teaching effort and expertise comes in a variety of forms, including formal feedback from learners, local and regional teaching awards, and invitations to teach from other services or schools. Each of these acknowledgments constitutes a data point in your case for promotion.

Education initiatives are welcome additions at teaching hospitals, whether with medical students, residents, fellows, or peers. Such projects enliven interactions and promote engagement by both teachers and learners. They may be cited as evidence of teaching excellence or leadership. Data on their effectiveness may be as simple as a satisfaction survey from participants, before and after test results, or broader measures of the program's success such as improved performance of trainees or increased recruitment of students into the field. Such projects may be recognized in their own right with awards or other acknowledgment, or they may be material for publication or dissemination through other means. They are concrete evidence of progress toward promotion.

Leadership

Administrative roles are essential in both academic and community-based settings and provide a variety of opportunities to develop and exercise leadership skills. Care teams have directors, clinical services have chiefs, departments have chairs, and hospitals have executives. Names and organizational structures vary, but the concepts of decision-making authority and accountability are consistent. These roles may or may not be desirable to you, but they are a reality of life in an institutional setting. Your choice of a hospital-based career is a tacit acknowledgment of your acceptance of work within a highly structured environment. Your willingness not only to tolerate that setting but also to contribute to its vision, methods, and effectiveness will determine how much to involve yourself in leadership roles. Your personal goals will set the degree to which this is part of your career aspirations and development. Specifics of leadership and administration are addressed in Chapter 6, "Leadership and Administration."

Vignette

Dr. G was excited to accept a clinical track appointment at her medical school and enthusiastically developed relationships with several senior faculty members as mentors in research and education. Her mentors noted, however, that despite her energy and stated interest in a series of projects that would facilitate her promotion to associate professor, her progress was slow and generally required significant intervention to come to fruition. Her academic trajectory seemed blocked, much to her and everyone else's frustration. The solution was finally identified with the retirement of her immediate superior on the hospital service. Moving into the role, Dr. G suddenly blossomed as an active, insightful, and decisive leader who effortlessly took on this responsibility. Within a short time, she had moved several steps up the administrative ladder, finding leadership a steady source of personal satisfaction and a platform for constructive action.

KEY POINTS

- Job satisfaction in the hospital environment requires comfort with routines, opportunities to develop skills and expertise, and a clear sense of purpose.

- Positive factors in maintaining well-being include the ability to find satisfaction in hospital-based clinical work, some degree of control over the work environment, and a sense of autonomy in daily decision-making.

- Risk for burnout should be monitored and addressed with modification of the work, social support, and professional interventions.

- Professional growth may take the form of skill development, formal promotion, or acceptance of leadership roles.

- Ready opportunities for academic activity include publication on topics routinely addressed on hospital services, use of clinical records for research projects, and development of teaching tools for trainees.

CHAPTER 6
Leadership and Administration

Laura Hirshbein, M.D., Ph.D.
Bradley Stilger, M.D.

In a famous scene in the middle
of the iconic film *The Snake Pit* (1948), the hero of the story, Dr. Kik, advocates for more time to work with his patient on a psychoanalytic revelation of her unconscious conflicts. His medical director counters Dr. Kik's passion for this individual patient by giving him statistics: overcrowding in every ward, admissions turned away, and demand from the community and from other hospitals. Dr. Kik insists that he needs to help his one patient. His medical director points out that they have an obligation to see the bigger picture. The film provides a fascinating look at the myriad treatments in psychiatry in the middle of the twentieth century, most of which are no longer in use. But this potential conflict between an individual patient–centered view and the perspective of an administrator still rings true.

Leadership within medical care requires a systems-level view. The needs of an individual patient must be balanced against the needs of the milieu (in a psychiatric inpatient unit), the resources of the hospital, and the

79

capacities of the staff. Those who take on administrative roles are often confronted by passionate advocates who want to make sure their individual patient gets optimal treatment. A leader needs to understand the systems, how they work together, and when and how to set limits on the demand for psychiatric services in a hospital, as well as be ready to master (or even better, work with people who have already mastered) issues around finances, regulation, and human resources across multiple disciplines.

Hospital-based psychiatry has always involved administrative roles for which most clinicians are not trained. These roles often have been accompanied by pressure to meet external demands and vulnerability to criticism. Even though there have long been challenges to figure out how to manage psychiatric systems, for better or worse, in the last few decades, medicine has moved toward a business model. Training in management is available to physicians and other health care leaders, but the approach, language, and principles are quite different from the clinical training that we receive to work with patients. This chapter makes no pretensions to offering business management guidance, nor does it try to take on the entire vast topic of administrative psychiatry. Instead, it represents lessons learned by physicians who have found themselves in leadership roles, as well as some guidance from published literature and reference sources. For more on this topic, see Talbott and Hales (2001) and Sharfstein et al. (2009).

What Systems Do You Have?

Psychiatric inpatient units are only one type of hospitalist-based service within a hospitalist model. Others include consultation-liaison services, psychiatric emergency evaluations, electroconvulsive therapy (ECT) services, and partial (day) hospital programs. Hospitals can be private, part of big health systems or academic medical centers, or sometimes a hybrid of multiple types. One of your challenges in administration of a hospital setting is understanding the organizational chart for the whole institution and where your institution fits into the bigger health system in the area. Where does your psychiatric service fit into the bigger picture? Do you report to your department? The hospital? Both? Where are the constraints on your hospital administrators? Are policies and procedures determined by each individual hospital or department or by business systems far outside the sites of patient care?

What is the scope of your administrative role? Are you responsible for the people? The space? The service utilization? The patient flow? What is the best way to interact with the rich complexity of services in most hospitals; for instance, how do you solve problems with dietary services or phlebotomy? How about housekeeping or facilities? And some of the psychiatry systems will intersect with different elements of the hospital. For example, psychiatry consultation services engage with medical-surgical teams, and psychiatric emergency services could be part of the general emergency department, a pediatric emergency department, or specialized psychiatric emergency services.

Inpatient Services

Psychiatric inpatient units can be located within a general hospital or as free-standing institutions, some of which have relationships with general hospitals. Both types of psychiatric hospitals are subject to specific laws governing admission and treatment based on the state where the hospital is located. The existence of this law and the complexity of administration within the hospital are often points of misunderstanding or conflict with general hospital administrators who do not understand that it is not possible to admit patients to a psychiatric space the same way that physicians admit to a medical-surgical service. It is essential for the medical director of a psychiatric unit to be fully conversant with the state laws regarding civil commitment. Hospital attorneys can often be helpful in clarifying elements of the law, but it is unlikely that an attorney will always be available to address routine questions, and physician leaders in other parts of the hospital system will want to be able to hear information from physician leadership in psychiatry. (Lawyer jokes aside, physicians do best hearing from other physicians.)

It is important that you have a clear understanding of the capabilities of the unit both from a space point of view and from a staffing perspective. Unlike medical-surgical hospitalization, patients in psychiatric hospitals can—and should—stay out of their rooms and interact with the staff and one another. Although the concept of a "therapeutic milieu" is somewhat old-fashioned (at least from a physician point of view), it is still highly relevant. Not all beds on an inpatient unit are the same. Some units have more secure spaces for agitated patients or patients who cannot be redirected. Most units have a combination of single rooms and double rooms (or rooms with even more beds). The task of filling all of the beds with the right combination of patients to provide a safe environment is difficult. It is also critical to have a process to get patients ready for discharge. What are the referral options in the area? The time immediately after discharge is the highest risk for suicidal patients. What are the follow-up options for patients who are discharged?

Inpatient units for children and adolescents can be especially challenging to set up and operate. Child psychiatry has always been a field with increasing demand and a shortage of providers, and that trend worsens every year. The potential patient populations for a child and adolescent unit can be extraordinarily diverse in terms of age and presenting problem. Nationally, relatively few inpatient psychiatric beds have been dedicated to pediatric populations, and it is challenging to get state approval to build more (for the many states that still operate under Certificate of Need guidelines). For existing units, hospital leaders have to make important decisions about how to manage demand, how to prioritize admissions, how (or whether) to handle high-acuity populations such as individuals with severe developmental disabilities, and how to incorporate families into treatment.

Consultation-Liaison Services

Psychiatry consultation teams are a valuable resource for medical-surgical services, but you may find it challenging to determine the appropriate staffing level for consultation services, as well as psychiatric emergency services, because the volume of requests can vary widely depending on the time of day, the part of the week, or the month of the year (and the variance is usually unpredictable). This is an advantage for hospitalist practice in that a dedicated cadre of staff members can be deployed as needed across a variety of hospital services if cross-training is provided for all of the services. Psychiatrists are key members of the consultation team, but it is also valuable to have advanced practice providers who can assist with typical questions around routine mental health care for medically hospitalized patients. Psychiatrically informed nurses or advanced practice providers can liaison with medical-surgical teams to assist them with key behavior strategies for challenging patients. Not all patients who become agitated, aggressive, or difficult to manage need to be on a psychiatry unit. Assistance personnel can help manage the anxiety and distress of medical-surgical teams that are overwhelmed with patient behaviors or symptoms. Social workers are likewise key members of consultation teams because they can not only engage in counseling but also assist with family communications or facilitate transfers to psychiatric units for the appropriate patients.

Much of your role as director of a consultation-liaison service will be managing the interactions between your staff and the consulting services. Physicians in every field experience increased anxiety and uncertainty with unfamiliar symptoms and diagnoses. Even the nature of the question being asked by the medical-surgical team may be a source of confusion or contention. A surgeon may rightly be convinced that disorientation and visual hallucinations should not occur on a surgery unit, but is the question one of diagnosis and treatment or one of service assignment and transfer? Is the primary task to clarify the medical issue or to educate the consulting service? As a leader managing a consultation service, make sure that your teams are diplomatic and good communicators, with a clear line for escalation of their concerns for your nonpsychiatric colleagues who have strong views about the mental health needs of their patients that may not match the expert opinions of the psychiatric consultants. As questions rise up the chain of command, make sure that you are familiar enough with the frontline operation of the service to appropriately respond.

Emergency Services

Psychiatric emergency services are critical within any hospital to handle the myriad behavioral emergencies that present. Most hospitals employ consultants to general emergency departments. For this model, as with the psychiatry consultation services for medical-surgical services, staffing needs to be flexible to handle variable demand. Some systems use well-trained social workers working alongside emergency department physicians to help guide decisions about admission to psychiatric inpatient units. Other systems have psychiatrists available some of the time rather than 24 hours a day. It could be reasonable to train emergency department advanced practice providers to do more psychiatric assessment. Regardless of the individuals involved, it is ideal to ensure that the focus remains a consideration of the patient's presentation and a matching between the patient's need and the appropriate level of care.

Set expectations for both hospital administration and patients about what an emergency psychiatric assessment will include. At a minimum, this will involve a brief history, bedside mental status examination, assessment of suicide or other risk, provisional diagnosis, recommendation for treatment or other follow-up, and clear documentation. Make sure that staff are appropriately trained in each of these tasks and held accountable for their completion.

If a hospital system does not have the resources to begin outpatient treatment for patients coming in for emergencies, it is important to create a robust system for referrals. As with general medicine, emergency assessments for behavioral health do not typically result in a cure or elimination of risk, a point often missed by patients, medical services, and higher-level administration. Similarly, not all patients who present can or should be hospitalized. Sometimes, despite the best efforts of expert clinicians, tragic outcomes still happen. Hospital administrators who understand the role and limitations of psychiatric emergency services will be most supportive with appropriate resources and responses to adverse events.

Ensure that your emergency service has appropriate access to security personnel and training in verbal and physical de-escalation for all staff. Nationwide, the highest incidence of assaults on staff occurs in emergency settings, both medical and psychiatric. To guarantee the immediate safety of patients and staff, security services must be readily available to help with physical management of agitated or aggressive patients. Security personnel also may assist by training staff members about nonviolent prevention of escalation and recognition of dangerous situations. This resource can be shared across the hospital system.

Other Services

Electroconvulsive Therapy

ECT requires collaboration between psychiatry and anesthesia and is most efficiently and safely conducted in a setting in which medical care is available in case of issues such as uncontrolled hypertension or delirium. Many patients who are undergoing ECT are psychiatrically hospitalized, so it is logical to locate the ECT program in close proximity to the psychiatric inpatient unit. The space to conduct ECT needs to be adequate for the service and take into consideration whether patients are coming from home for treatments or from the hospital.

Partial Hospital Programs

Partial hospital programs can bridge the gap between the psychiatric inpatient unit and ambulatory care but are only viable in settings with a high demand for hospital services. Carefully examine the needs of your community, payer mix, and legal requirements for the program. The location of a partial hospital program near the inpatient unit (and staffed with hospitalist personnel) can help manage a higher-acuity patient population, provide adequate staffing as the census fluctuates, and allow sharing of ancillary personnel such as activity therapists and social workers.

Development of New Systems

Development of new systems can be an exciting element of administration and leadership. As awareness of mental health issues increases around the United States, high-level hospital administrators are more willing to devote resources to behavioral health. Although most mental health hospital services are not well reimbursed (other than ECT), dedicated behavioral health services are a benefit to a general hospital, and expanded service options are invaluable for free-standing psychiatric hospitals. Some health systems are eager to try to tackle some of the hardest patient populations to manage, such as substance-abusing patients or individuals with severe intellectual disabilities. Other systems are excited about the potential for innovative biomedical interventions (new treatments such as transcranial magnetic stimulation or ketamine). Pitching a new system will require you to demonstrate that staffing is feasible and that there is value—financially or from a patient care perspective—to the institution.

Who Do You Have to Work With? Interdisciplinary Systems

Vignette

A group of academic physicians in a large community practice setting had a traditional model for their practice, which meant that they were expected to manage ongoing outpatient clinics during most of the year except for 1–2 months when they were expected to attend on the inpatient unit. Some faculty appreciated the opportunity to care for the higher-acuity patients, whereas others were resentful of the need to choose between putting their clinics on hold and trying to see both inpatients and outpatients in a busy day. There were not enough residents in the training program to cover the inpatient unit. The faculty group discussed two different pilot models: one would split the faculty into outpatient and hospitalist, and the other would hire and train a cadre of advanced practice providers to do the primary management of patients in the hospital so that the faculty could be more focused during their times on the hospital service. They found that faculty were divided, depending on where and how they wanted to spend their time; some wanted a higher-level overview perspective and liked the prospect of having advanced practice providers manage the details, but others wanted to go more in-depth with patients in one setting.

In an ideal world, it should be possible to match up an individual's training, role in a health system, and key strengths to maximize everyone's success. Hospital settings are not for everyone. Patients can be challenging from the perspective of medical acuity, personality organization, or intensity of external problems. Some physicians are more comfortable with patients who can talk through problems, whereas others prefer more of a crisis focus in their interactions. Other kinds of hospital staff members are critical to effective maintenance of therapeutic environments. When considering hospital team structures, we have to look at the roles of the different disciplines and the passions and strengths of the individuals involved.

Psychiatrists

Physicians are obviously key personnel for psychiatric services. In many hospitals, psychiatrists are not devoted full time to these programs. Some organizations employ psychiatrists who are in clinic for part of the day and come to the hospital only in the morning or the evening. Some spread their inpatient staff to see consultations and psychiatric emergencies. From an administrative point of view, however, it is much easier to have a dedicated hospitalist staff whose first priority is the high-acuity space. Furthermore, it is significantly easier to manage problem solving with a smaller number of dedicated faculty who are familiar to the other services. Physicians are really the only discipline for which there is a possibility of being detailed outside the hospital setting. If physicians are divided among locations, especially with different administrative structures, it is imperative to have clear expectations for both the physician and the clinical service about priorities and time.

Physician Quality Improvement

Physician quality improvement can be a challenging issue. Today's medical environment has increasing focus on assurance of high-quality care and measurement of outcomes. These are difficult to do with psychiatrists, however, especially in the hospital setting. Patients are often upset about being in the hospital; sometimes they are involuntary and want to leave, and sometimes they have personality disturbances and do not want to be discharged. Patient opinion about their providers may reflect more about the patients and less about the providers. Furthermore, recovery in the hospital is a function of the whole staff rather than the provider, and that itself is difficult to quantify. More challenging still, physicians are traditionally independent in their interactions with their patients (after residency training), so it is unclear when, why, or how a supervisor could or should intervene with physician practice.

From a basic quality perspective, it is reasonable to conduct routine audits of documentation of patient care by physicians. For psychiatric encounters, certain elements of the documentation should be present, including a suicide risk assessment, the diagnosis, and the treatment plan. Part of your responsibility is to set expectations about chart audits and establish a mechanism for review with the physician and remediation if needed. It is reasonable to survey staff members who work with the physician (as should probably be the case in each discipline) to elicit feedback about the work environment. A useful practice is to formalize these surveys and to make them anonymous so that staff have no fear of reprisal if they make a negative comment. Again, it is important to set an expectation with the physician that these surveys are part of employment (perhaps in a yearly performance evaluation).

Role Selection

Role selection within hospital settings includes consideration of intensity, predictability, and degree of interaction with other specialties. This can be challenging for a variety of reasons. Your selection of staff for hospital roles should take into account the provider's temperament, skills at diplomacy, communication abilities, and response to pressure. From a leader's perspective, things run most smoothly when physicians are a good fit for their practice environment, not just in a role that needed to be filled or the environment they prefer.

Advanced Practice Providers

Advanced practice providers include both nurse practitioners and physician assistants. These providers can be extremely helpful in extending physician reach in terms of prescribing, quality time with patients, and communication with other members of the teams. Nationally, there has been fear that advanced practice providers will be hired in place of psychiatrists and that physician job security is at risk. These fears have interfered with good relationships with psychiatrists in many states. The reality is, however, that there is such a high degree of need for mental health services that adding advanced practice providers most likely will not diminish the need for psychiatrists. Instead, psychiatrists can devote more time and energy to the highly complex patients, while advanced practice providers can assist with those challenging patients or manage more straightforward cases. From a patient point of view, a well-trained individual who is ready to engage with him or her is invaluable.

Challenges you will face with advanced practice providers include understanding union regulations (for nurse practitioners), scope of practice guidelines (depending on the state), issues with mental health law (whether advanced practice providers complete civil commitment paperwork, for example), and training. The last issue is particularly key. Advanced practice providers do not have the same kind of training within systems that is done by medical students. As a result, advanced practice providers may have gaps in knowledge about how the medical system works and also may have limitations in expertise in some areas. Collaboration with advanced practice providers works best when they are treated as professionals who want to learn and grow in their field. They should be given adequate training in psychopharmacology, basic modalities of therapy, and insights into diagnostic practices at a minimum. Advanced practice providers also can be trained to function within ECT programs and in all areas of hospital practice.

Nurses

Nursing is the central discipline within any inpatient unit and is critical to the quality of a clinical program. Nursing is highly structured and functions within a tighter chain of command than most physicians are accustomed to. Furthermore, there is a push within nursing to familiarize nurses with the published literature and to engage in evidence-based nursing practice. In broad strokes, nurses follow physician orders, but nurses are trained to use their own skills and not just blindly follow orders. Physicians make diagnoses and treatment plans, and nurses implement those plans but have significant leeway to make adjustments in response to patients' preferences, degree of cooperation, and behaviors. Far from passive conduits of treatment, they are highly interactive with patients, allowing them to make subtle, long-term, and detailed observations and to establish strong working relationships with patients and families. Metaphorically, patients are on a journey to wellness, physicians identify the destination and select the route, and nurses drive the bus; each role is essential.

From an administrative point of view, it is critical that you have a productive working relationship with nursing leadership. For psychiatric inpatient unit management, the ideal is a partnership between the medical director and the nurse manager. As medical director, you will likely not have time (or expertise) to address the minutia of nursing practice but will need to understand how to make adjustments in practice to best meet the needs of the patients and staff. A good relationship with a nurse manager can help you learn more about nursing culture and practice and problem solve when issues arise. The nurses are managing the day-to-day environment on the unit, as well as the patient flow around activities. High-quality nursing is often the difference between an adequate unit and an outstanding unit. Nurses can also be key partners in psychiatry consultation settings, either on medical-surgical floors or in emergency departments. General nurses in those areas often respond best to a well-trained psychiatric nurse, and they can collaborate on problem solving within the nursing scope of practice.

Social Workers

Social work is a major partner in psychiatric hospital settings. To a greater degree than other disciplines, the scope of social work practice can vary widely depending on the demands of the system and the skills of the social worker. Some social workers are primarily trained to help patients with systems issues, including accessing outpatient resources or transferring patients to inpatient units. Other social workers have training in family systems and can be invaluable assets for inpatient teams who want to enhance their engagement with patients' support systems during a hospitalization. Some social workers are trained as therapists for individual or group work and can do brief therapy interventions for patients in a hospital setting.

One of your challenges in a hospital setting is determining where social workers fit into the chain of command. Should they report to the physicians? The nurses? Higher-level administrators? Social work leadership? No clear answer is available, leaving a measure of ambiguity regarding their working relationship with other disciplines and accountability for their work. Unfortunately, despite their tremendous value for patient care, transitions of care, and family systems, social workers are often underpaid and underappreciated. As with any discipline, the skill and dedication of individual social workers are as important as the particular task assigned in determining their true value.

Activity Therapists

Activity therapy is an important element of inpatient care, often making the difference between a well-regarded, therapeutically valuable psychiatric inpatient unit and a primarily custodial environment. Various subspecialties exist within activity therapy, including recreational therapy, music therapy, and occupational therapy. Each of these therapists is specially licensed to do group and individual work with adults and children on inpatient units. For many systems, they provide the bulk of activities to occupy patients' time while in the hospital. Their services can be mobilized to support patients on the medical-surgical floors who could benefit from additional services dedicated to mental health. It makes sense to align inpatient unit activity therapy strengths with the goals and priorities of the unit. If an inpatient unit wants to focus on dialectical behavior therapy (DBT), for example, it would be logical to recruit or train activity therapists who could incorporate the DBT skills into activities for the patients. Conversely, if a unit has a particular strength in one area from dedicated activity therapists, it might make sense to prioritize patients who could benefit from that service.

Psychologists and Teachers

Psychologists and teachers are especially valuable for child and adolescent inpatient units. As with social workers, psychologists can vary widely in their scope of interest and practice, from testing to structured behavioral interventions to general psychotherapy. Although formal psychological testing is not necessarily indicated for routine hospital-based services, it can be valuable to differentiate among diagnostic possibilities for some confusing or complex patients. Testing is also helpful for a baseline for patients about to undergo ECT or for children who are having academic difficulties. For children and adolescents who are psychiatrically hospitalized, it is critical to have educational specialists who can assess the patients, coordinate with their teachers and schools, and support the students' ongoing education.

Team Communication and Meetings

Regardless of the discipline and the service, a critical element of psychiatric work is in team collaboration. Electronic medical record (EMR) systems are used by health systems partly as a form of communication, but as many people have found over the last decade of advancement in EMRs, the electronic record cannot substitute for face-to-face team communications. Many EMR systems compartmentalize information or create separate portal systems for different disciplines. Others contain so much information that it is easy to get lost. All of the EMRs run the risk of putting the computer rather than the patient at the center of health care. Team meetings, as old-fashioned as they may seem, continue to provide important venues for the different disciplines to come together, understand what is happening with a patient, share information, and make a plan going forward. Although each service will have to balance team meeting time with the obligations of direct patient care, a reasonable amount of time in team collaboration is well spent in terms of cohesiveness of team interactions with patients, problem solving around difficult issues, and management of milieu concerns.

Vignette

A busy hospital psychiatric emergency service was staffed with social workers and physicians. Everyone seemed to be working all the time, and the patients kept flooding the system. Everything seemed to take forever. The emergency system administrator embarked on the difficult task of trying to recruit new faculty to staff the service. More patients, he reasoned, meant that more psychiatrists would be needed. The senior administrator in the department, however, took a step back and looked at all the tasks that had to be accomplished and the ideal individual for each task. She was able to determine that patients would flow through the system more quickly with more nurses who could triage, social workers who could focus on facilitating disposition, and the same number of physicians who could more easily focus on assessments and plans.

Patient care is complex and involves many moving parts. Although it is clear that each discipline involved with patients has a different role, it is less clear in any particular setting who should be doing what. Sometimes systems evolve over time, and it becomes tradition, rather than scope of practice, that determines who gets basic information from the patient (including medications, allergies, psychiatric history, medical history, social history, substance abuse history), who talks to the family, who completes physical examinations if needed, who coordinates care with outpatient providers, and who documents. Many systems involve redundant efforts; both nurses and physicians, for example, may document medical history. Efficiency can certainly be an overworked concept; only so many things can be streamlined or cut from practice. But examining duplication or inefficiencies in workflow can definitely make a difference when making staffing decisions.

What Can You Do? Patient Flow and Strategic Choices

Vignette

The medical director of an inpatient unit received a call from a major researcher within his department. The researcher said that he had a patient coming to the hospital's emergency department, and he wanted to ensure that the patient would make it onto the hospital's inpatient unit. The medical director heard about the case—a young woman with severe anorexia and intense self-harm behaviors—and worried that his unit would not be able to handle the patient's acuity or behaviors. When he shared this with the researcher, the researcher said that the patient's family was a major donor to his research program. Furthermore, the researcher suggested that if the medical director refused, he would involve the chair of the department.

One of the greatest challenges you will face as medical director of a psychiatric service is to manage the demand for care in an environment that does not have enough providers, beds in psychiatric hospitals, or referral opportunities to meet demand. There is a robust literature about the issues of psychiatric beds and of whether there are enough from a policy point of view. But in this area, a policy perspective comes up hard against the expectations and demands of any given patient, family, or highly placed individual within the system. It is understandable that family members and patients would be focused on the unique needs of their one psychiatric patient. Sometimes providers become equally passionate that it is essential to accommodate the patient they have in front of them, regardless of how complex or whether he or she could benefit the most or is the highest priority for the psychiatric services.

It is important for you to have a clear idea of the mission of an inpatient unit. Not all units have the same strengths or capacities. What can the staff do well? What are the facilities set up to provide, or what are the limitations of the physical layout of the unit? If the inpatient unit has mostly double rooms (or larger) with a great deal of open space, it will be harder to treat acute patients because the milieu will be more interactive (and therefore harder to manage). On the contrary, if an inpatient unit has several staff who are trained in a particular kind of therapy or intervention, then the unit could focus on that issue. Some challenging patient populations include aggressive or impulsive individuals, those with severe self-harm behaviors, those with behavior disturbances (such as eating disorders, brain injuries, or autism spectrum disorders), and those with complex medical issues or dementia. Does the inpatient unit have a responsibility to serve a particular area around the hospital or a specific clinic? If you clearly articulate what the unit can do well—and, conversely, what the unit is unable to do well—it will help to address this challenge.

It is critical to coordinate hospital services to organize patient flow and priorities. If patients are admitted to the inpatient service from an emergency department as well as from a medical-surgical service (after being seen by a psychiatry consultant), which patients should take priority if there are not enough beds to accommodate everyone? What other services or hospitals are available in the community that could serve as alternatives to the hospital? What is the process by which patients are assessed for admission to the inpatient unit? Who makes those decisions? What issues belong to nursing, and which belong to physicians?

Patients with medical comorbidities, including issues such as alcohol withdrawal, can present additional challenges. For units in general hospitals, you must be able to identify adequate medical consultation. Educate those consultants to the ways that psychiatry is not like other units in the hospital. Patients are typically ambulatory within the unit, not lying in beds. Psychiatric nurses function differently from medical-surgical nurses. You will need to communicate clearly with the consulting services about what issues must be managed by the consultants and what can be done by the primary team. In deciding whether a patient can be managed on a psychiatry unit or must remain on (or go to) a medical floor, nursing capacities and competencies need to be considered. Be clear about what is needed to ensure that psychiatric patients stay safe.

For all psychiatric units, it is necessary to have a sense of what kinds of medical comorbidities can be managed on the unit. True medical-psychiatric units are relatively uncommon, but most psychiatric units within general hospitals can tolerate some degree of medical comorbidity. Articulate with staff what kinds of medical issues will never be accepted on inpatient psychiatry units (such as patients on ventilators) versus medical care that might be possible with additional training for staff. Clarify with hospital administration whether a medical consultant to a psychiatric unit is responsible for direct patient care, writing orders, and directing nursing, or if a consultant is advising the primary psychiatric team. Have a clear pathway to quickly escalate decision-making if patient safety is at risk.

Carefully articulate with admitting services the goals and limitations of a psychiatric hospitalization. Make sure that everyone involved in admission decisions is sharing those with patients and families. On consultation-liaison services, educate medical-surgical teams about the expected benefits and limitations of a psychiatric intervention. Good diplomacy and clear communication are essential in consultation and emergency services.

For the inpatient team, make sure that the entire staff is aligned with the purpose and function of the hospitalization. Interdisciplinary staff events are useful mechanisms to ensure that everyone appreciates the shared vision. Patients notice when they are getting different messages from different disciplines about their care, and that inconsistency is noted in patient satisfaction data. Although it is certainly not possible to please all patients and meet all of their needs in an acute hospitalization, it is reasonable to set goals with a consistent tone throughout the staff. Tight coordination, shared responsibility, and clear communication among leaders of the different disciplines can help to set standards so patients and staff members know what to expect.

One of the areas that is the most difficult to manage on the unit is patient flow outward. It is a risky proposition to discharge many patients, especially those with unstable home situations or who had been threatening suicide. However, hospitalization can have diminishing benefits for patients who will have to return to their usual environment at some point. A prolonged hospitalization can diminish their ability to function, regress their coping skills, and increase the contrast between being cared for in the hospital and their regular lives. Several things can help both patients and staff members with the discharge process.

Establish an expectation for your staff of clear goals and expectations for the purpose of the hospital stay. Although the hospital is a refuge, it is also a treatment environment, and activities and things must be accomplished. Begin talking about discharge from the time of admission, and set the expectation right away that one of the goals of the hospital stay is to prepare to leave. This allows the patient to partner with staff to identify barriers to discharge, address problems that need to be resolved or mitigated before discharge, and articulate needs that must be addressed. Furthermore, beginning a conversation about discharge allows both the patient and the staff a sense of control and direction of the process. Patients are part of the decision-making about discharge, and their sense of agency is reinforced. For staff members who are frustrated with a patient or who have trouble letting go, a plan for discharge gives them an exit strategy. Discharge planning involves every member of the staff, from the physician to the nurse to the activity therapist to the social worker. To eliminate confusion for the patient, staff members from the different disciplines must be clear and consistent. Messaging to the patient needs to be unified and convey that the patient is developing the tools required to get ready for discharge. A central tracking tool, whether in the EMR or on a nursing station board, can be helpful to ensure that everyone is on the same page.

Put procedures in place to manage the ongoing challenge of high-risk discharges. Confirm the availability of bridging appointments within a day or two after discharge to ensure continuity of care so that those patients are seen. Involve a process of follow-up telephone calls. Find available step-down care through a high-quality partial hospital program. Expect reports from staff on whether these patients met with their next-care providers and the steps they took if that handoff failed.

What Do You Need to Avoid? Regulatory Systems and Legal Issues

Regulatory Systems

Regulatory systems are intended to ensure that hospitals meet an adequate threshold for patient safety. You will likely interface with various regulatory agencies depending on level of care and region. Common agencies include The Joint Commission, Centers for Medicare and Medicaid Services (CMS), and state mental health agencies. Many institutions have specific departments meant to focus on maintenance of accreditation, but it is important for you to have a working knowledge of the standards and expectations relevant to your area. These standards are always evolving, and it may take a concerted effort to stay aware of recent information and recommendations.

A site visit or review by an accrediting agency can be a source of anxiety for any administrative team, regardless of how seasoned or prepared you may be. The sight of The Joint Commission surveyor may send even the most seasoned leaders into hiding. During site visits, it is critical to stay calm, have ready access to your policies and procedures, and be concise in answering the surveyors' questions. Focus on showing them exactly what they ask for and need to know—too much obfuscation can lead to confusion (and citations). Maintain an air of transparency, but be concise. If possible, have leadership from multiple disciplines available for clarification of specific points.

Facilities and Environment

Facilities concerns are often a headache for psychiatric administrators. Although psychiatry is a relatively low-technology specialty, the minimal equipment involved, such as a hospital bed, generates an inordinate amount of discussion and anxiety. There has been national concern about the effect of the physical environment on patient safety. Regulatory agencies such as The Joint Commission have focused recent surveys on aspects of the environment that pose a potential risk for self-harm, particularly hanging. Surveyors inspect beds, bathroom fixtures, and even gaps around picture frames. Their presence is a reminder that you are responsible for more than just your staff's active work with patients.

Malpractice Suits

Your awareness of patient safety, both during and after their stays, may help you deal with a reasonable fear of lawsuits. Physicians fear discharging high-risk patients because their vulnerability to legal action exceeds their capacity to predict behavior. Nurses hear horror stories of lawsuits by patients who fall and injure themselves. Clinicians within all disciplines, even unit clerks, walk the line between respecting patients' wishes for privacy and adequately collaborating with their families and other care providers.

Fear is not a good basis on which to practice medicine or maintain morale. It is an unfortunate reality that the dual burdens of predicting the future and controlling human behavior have been placed on our shoulders, when in reality we know just how little we can ultimately control. Help your staff stay focused on doing their best work, meeting the standard of care, and recognizing the limits of interventions. Provide prompt debriefing under quality assurance protections for staff involved in an adverse event. Continue to offer nonjudgmental support throughout any review, investigative, or legal process.

How Can You Keep the Lights On? Finances, Billing, and Budgets

The reality of monetary considerations in medicine is as inevitable as it is unfortunate. Whatever humanist motives and altruistic intentions you harbor, nearly all health care ultimately requires a firm financial footing to en-sure its continuity. Your role as a leader and administrator requires you to keep an eye on those issues. Unlike some private practices or outpatient of-fices, hospital services are rarely stand-alone entities but rather are part of larger financial structures. Thus, budgets are not generally about matching revenues to expenditures but rather matching performance to expectations. Budgets become matters of negotiation over issues such as facility charges, support staff, and institutional goals, informed by realities of patient popu-lation and reimbursement models.

Budget Negotiations

Psychiatry is a time-intensive specialty whose services are undervalued relative to other aspects of medical care. This is particularly true in hospital settings where patient acuity is high and intensive services need to be brought to bear quickly. Emergency and consultation services typically require full staffing at all times to handle intermittent and unpredictable times of high demand. Con-sultation services are invariably subject to low reimbursement rates. Inpatient services are under constant pressure to minimize hospital days and are at the mercy of payer assessment as to whether care provided was "medically neces-sary," often determined by a nonmedical professional and invariably reviewed by an individual without direct access to the patient. Consequently, these ser-vices will not be profit centers for most hospitals and typically have to be sub-sidized by more lucrative procedure-based specialties.

Hospitals include mental health facilities because they want those services for their patients and the welfare of the community, they save money for other clinical specialties, and some regulatory bodies require them. Thus, the value of psychiatry is not fully measured by its revenues but by its effect on the wel-fare of patients and the overall operation of the medical center. Although it can be difficult to place a monetary value on those factors, it is essential.

Keep all of these issues in mind as you enter negotiations with your medical center administration. Insist on a clear message about what services the insti-tution needs and expects. Be clear about the cost of those services, and provide realistic expectations for reimbursement. Anticipate reasonable pushback re-garding performance variables such as patient flow and reimbursement levels. Do frequent reality checks with your own expectations and those of the insti-tution to ensure that your service can actually deliver whatever you agree to.

Efficiency and Revenue Optimization

Although hospital services may not be profitable, their bottom line can be improved by consistent attention to how services are organized, documented, and billed. Devote time to regular reviews of patient flow—to how long it takes to provide appropriate care, how much time the patient and staff spend waiting for things, and how quickly the patient can be returned to the outpatient setting. Look for ways to perform these tasks more efficiently. Avoid duplication of effort. Identify recurrent causes of unnecessary delay and seek to address them.

Use staff efficiently. Make sure that staff members are working at the upper range of their skill sets. In large clinical operations, allow clerical staff to gather demographic information, check insurance coverage, and complete paperwork. Have social workers contact family and outside providers and gather social and family history. Nurses can assess and triage patients, administer medications, and monitor medical issues. Limit physician activity to formal assessment, treatment planning, and required documentation. In smaller settings, where services are inactive between busy periods, find other useful tasks for them to do, possibly covering more than one service.

Maximize billing for appropriate services whenever possible. All too often, legitimately billable service goes uncompensated because of inadequate documentation. Use templates and flags in EMRs to remind physicians of key elements and phrases in notes. Arrange regular training and frequent feedback on documentation for billing purposes. Payer liaison staff are skilled at identifying the key phrases that payers use to determine medical necessity and level of care for patients. They should share those with note writers and give them immediate feedback on how services are being billed and why. Make sure that your staff are getting paid for the services they are performing.

Vignette

The newly hired attending on a busy inpatient service quickly developed a reputation for thorough clinical care, efficient work habits, and excellent relationships with patients and families but was taken aback at her annual review to have a below-standard score on patient reimbursement. This was never part of her residency training, and she considered her succinct, focused notes to be a source of pride and mark of clinical maturity. A specialist from the payer liaison office took the time to sit down with her and review each of the elements of her notes. With that feedback, she began to replace phrases such as "Denied medication side effects" with "Denied rigidity, sedation, and constipation." "Discussed discharge with patient and family" gave way to "Held 35-minute family meeting before discharge." Co-signatures on house officer notes were now accompanied by a "pull-down" attestation that she was present for the visit. This specification of systems reviewed and time actually spent on tasks required minimal extra effort but significantly increased reimbursement on her notes.

How Can You Make Things Better? Quality Improvement and Staff Wellness

Quality Improvement

Quality improvement, broadly defined as a data-driven approach to analyzing practice performance and informing practice change, has long been a challenge in psychiatry. Psychiatric diagnoses and outcomes are based on interpretation of patient reports that can be subjective and difficult to measure quantitatively. Despite these challenges, regulatory agencies continue to emphasize quality improvement across health care as a whole, and the field of psychiatry is not immune to this pressure. Increasingly, regulatory agencies are expecting clinics and institutions to report data metrics as a component of reimbursement and accreditation.

Your role in clinic administration includes responsibility for these issues. Look for quality improvement measures that assess compliance with expected regulations or standards of care, seek clear guidelines or algorithms to guide treatment practices, and implement measurements of psychiatric outcomes. Examples of measures could include percentage of patients with a diagnosis of depression for which a suicide risk assessment is completed, provider compliance with documentation of current medications, or percentage of patients who have had a risk assessment for falls. The American Psychiatric Association (2017) has compiled a list of measures that pertain to psychiatric practice, selected from the Merit-Based Incentive Payment System program measures published by Medicare and CMS. The Joint Commission has created a set of measures called the Hospital Based Inpatient Psychiatric Services Psychiatric Core Measures, meant to improve the quality and safety of patient care provided on psychiatric inpatient units. Examples of the core measures include admission screening for violence risk and psychological trauma, hours of physical restraint and seclusion use, and patients discharged on multiple antipsychotic medications with appropriate justification (Joint Commission 2019).

Patient Satisfaction

Assessment of how patients feel about hospital-based mental health care is complex and often ambiguous. Patients may have been treated involuntarily, expectations may have been unrealistic, or their perception of the treatment experience may have been distorted—all possible manifestations of the very illnesses for which they entered treatment and all of which would obviously influence any patient satisfaction measure. Not unexpectedly, little consensus exists regarding standard tools with which psychiatric patients' impressions should be measured, although many varied measurement tools do already exist in the literature (Miglietta et al. 2018). Your choice of survey instruments will depend on your goals in measuring satisfaction and may be specific to the treatments or programs being rendered. Some institutions choose to employ a third-party organization tasked with collecting and collating the patient satisfaction data, at higher cost but greater efficiency than many in-house processes.

Staff Wellness

Staff wellness has become the new aspiration for many health system administrators who recognize that employee burnout is an enormous problem for health care. At a minimum, ensure that your staff have access to an employee assistance program with adequate mental health services. Psychiatric patients manifest an extensive range of intense emotions, and staff may be overwhelmed by the secondary trauma of engaging with patients' stories of horrendous events, externalizing behaviors, and suicidal thoughts and behaviors. Perhaps even more valuable than offering access to services is promoting an environment in which all can feel that the burden is shared and that their strong reactions to patients are normal and expected.

To promote general wellness, many institutions are making more concerted efforts to integrate initiatives such as fitness programs and health education into employee culture. Although not necessarily specific to those working in the mental health field, these programs can help to promote or incentivize important aspects of general health and wellness. Groups on mindfulness, relaxation, and other coping skills are easy to organize, often appreciated by staff, and well worth the effort.

Conclusion

Administrative roles in hospital psychiatry can be challenging and rewarding. The acute nature of hospital care means that things are moving quickly and that patients are in crisis. The work is seldom boring but often demanding and draining. For leaders, the challenge is to build a system that balances the ability to respond to an issue in the moment (reaction) with the capacity to plan for improvement through clear and consistent policies for the future (proactive planning), while also balancing the needs and goals of individuals with those of the larger institution. This role is not for everyone, because it requires the capacity to empathize, strategize, compromise, and tolerate conflict in equal measure. It is both humbling and empowering, and for those who do it well, this role is satisfying and appreciated.

KEY POINTS

- Hospital systems as a whole and as individual services need to have a clear vision of the purpose of the service; the target patient population; and the methods for admission, treatment, and discharge.

- Hospital-based treatment requires well-functioning, multidisciplinary teams who communicate effectively both electronically and in team interactions.

- Systems need to be aligned so that patients can move smoothly from one to another as needed.

- Physician leaders need strong administrative partners to facilitate complex issues, especially around regulatory affairs.

- Administrators should manage the budget by realistic negotiation with medical center administration, efficient use of resources, and optimization of documentation for billing.

- Quality improvement and staff wellness are integral parts of any hospital system, with clear benefits for both care providers and patients.

References

American Psychiatric Association: Quality measures for 2017 MIPS quality category reporting. 2017. Available at: https://www.psychiatry.org/psychiatrists/practice/quality-improvement/quality-measures-for-mips-quality-category. Accessed February 4, 2020.

Joint Commission: Specifications Manual for Joint Commission National Quality Measures. August 1, 2019. Available at: https://manual.jointcommission.org/releases/TJC2020A. Accessed February 7, 2020.

Miglietta E, Belessiotis-Richards C, Ruggeri M, Priebe S: Scales for assessing patient satisfaction with mental health care: a systematic review. J Psychiatr Res 100:33–46, 2018 29482063

Sharfstein SS, Dickerson FB, Oldham JM (eds): Textbook of Hospital Psychiatry. Washington, DC, American Psychiatric Publishing, 2009

Talbott JA, Hales RE (eds): Textbook of Administrative Psychiatry: New Concepts for a Changing Behavioral Health System, 2nd Edition. Washington, DC, American Psychiatric Publishing, 2001

CHAPTER 7
Teaching and Supervision

Michael Casher, M.D.

The calling of the teacher. There is no craft more privileged. To
awaken in another human being powers, dreams beyond one's own; to
induce in others a love for that which one loves; to make of one's
inward present their future; that is a threefold adventure like no other.

George Steiner, Lessons of the Masters

Share your knowledge. It is a way to achieve immortality.

Dalai Lama XIV

In this chapter, I explore the
considerable teaching and supervisory roles for a psychiatric hospitalist.
Whether you are involved in consultation-liaison work, psychiatric emergency services work, or inpatient psychiatry, or even split your time among
these three main branches of hospital psychiatry, you will likely be called on
to teach and supervise in some capacity. As is clear from the other chapters
of this book, although some issues are specific to each of these settings, considerable overlap is seen in the patient populations and clinical dilemmas en-

demic to each of these specialized sites in psychiatry to the point that many hospitalists are comfortable in two or all three of these settings. In addition, whether one is in a university setting with a full-time position or working at a community hospital as a psychiatry attending who also has some responsibility for rotating residents and/or medical students, supervision and teaching will consume a certain percentage of time. Whether this pedagogic role becomes a joyful enterprise for you and, indeed, part of your calling as a physician or, conversely, an odious task that only adds to the burdens of clinical work depends on a host of factors, both distal and proximal to the immediate clinical situation. Your attitude toward and rapport with learners, your comfort in a teaching situation, and the skill with which you impart complex information will all be influenced by distal personal experiences with teachers and mentors (we should add parents here as well, as the process we are describing is largely one of modeling and identification). The quality and effectiveness of your teaching efforts will be fostered—or, conversely, hindered— "proximally" by the nature of the environment in which you are now working and attempting to inculcate your accumulated knowledge into the young minds of those trainees in your charge (for instance, is ample time allotted for teaching? Is the teaching role valued at your institution?).

Would that we all could achieve the Buddha-like beatific attitudes about teaching depicted in the opening quotes from George Steiner and the Dalai Lama! But it is feasible for most of us to improve our pedagogic skills by looking systematically at the elements of good teaching and supervision. In other words, we all need to make up for the deficit in most standard psychiatric trainings in which we learned a lot about psychodiagnosis, psychopharmacology, and various psychotherapies but had little or no formal instruction or supervision in how to teach. This chapter then is a humble attempt to address this gap by outlining common problems, issues, challenges, and opportunities that face a psychiatric hospitalist (and perhaps one who is relatively new to the position) with an interest in teaching and supervision and, in the process, to offer guidelines, pearls, strategies, and overall ways to conceptualize the supervisory or teaching endeavor. The hope is that this will offer a framework so that you can come up with your own solutions to the new problems that inevitably arise.

The pace of the work, the acuity of the patients, the variety of psychopathology, the opportunity to work with other medical and mental health disciplines—all of these elements combine to make the various psychiatric hospital settings premier places for learning. This is as true for psychiatry as it is for other medical disciplines, and for many of us, our most vivid recollections of our training—even years later—are of experiences with challenging patients "in extremis" in the hospital. Best is when whatever twinge of discomfort we feel with these recollections is tempered by an accompanying association to a helpful supervisor whose expertise, counsel, and availability saw us through the care of a given patient. The task of this chapter could rightfully be seen as addressing the following question: What are the attitudes, approaches, and methods that you should develop and foster in yourself as a teacher/supervisor so that you will be recalled in such a positive way by your learners when they look back at their training years?

Specific Characteristics of Teaching Psychiatry in the Hospital

Each of the three hospital psychiatry sectors has specific types of patients and clinical situations that will call forth your supervisory skills, and you should be prepared to explain your philosophy and clinical reasoning to different levels of learners for each of these variations. Inpatient work, for instance, will involve the short-term stabilization and management of acute psychiatric illnesses such as mania, acute psychotic states of the schizophrenia spectrum, refractory depression, and severe regressions in patients with borderline personality disorder. Your students and residents will have the opportunity to see progress in many of their patients in a short time (a great recruiting tool for psychiatry, by the way). Inpatient units offer the chance to supervise the care of major psychiatric illnesses in the acute phase and to teach (and this is just a short list, of course) acute use of psychopharmacological agents, management of agitation, indications for electroconvulsive therapy, criteria for discharge, working with a multidisciplinary team, and the legal issues involved in involuntary hospitalization.

Consultation-liaison psychiatry services will offer teaching opportunities that intersect with those on inpatient psychiatry to some extent, but with an added emphasis on detection and management of delirium, psychological responses to medical illness, the assessment of capacity, and the liaison with medical and surgical staff for management of "difficult" patients.

The psychiatric emergency department will be the most hectic and acute of all settings, with prototypical patients, for instance, brought in by first responders in an agitated psychotic state or transferred from a medical emergency department after medical clearance following an intentional overdose. The psychiatric emergency department is where residents particularly can learn how to do a thorough but focused evaluation that informs crucial decisions about admission versus the need for further workup or even acute management in the psychiatric emergency department. Supervision in the psychiatric emergency department, by nature of the pace of the work, will tend to be more "off-the-cuff," but your residents and, to some extent, the medical students can use this setting to learn how to do an incisive suicide risk assessment and how to assess whether a patient needs hospitalization against his or her will. Emergency psychiatry will give you the chance to show residents and students how to perform a templated mental status examination and how to review the laboratory tests essential in distinguishing medical causes of altered mental status (including psychosis) from primary psychiatric disorders, all of which is in the service of honing their acute clinical decision-making skills.

It is important for you to accommodate to how students and residents at different levels and from various disciplines will have different learning needs. The best teachers are those who are able to navigate the challenge on clinical rounds of keeping everyone interested and engaged even though different levels of learners are involved. Some attendings manage this by inserting pearl-like points into the discussion after each patient is seen and by fostering an inquisitive approach with a few pithy questions or comments. One nice pedagogic tool is to use the more senior residents to explain to the earlier learners the basic pathology and the treatment approach for a given patient and reserving your expertise for some "fine-tuning" comments or for summarizing the discussion. Keeping in mind the disparate levels of learners (and perhaps related disciplines who may also be present) and making teaching comments that everyone can use will win respect and foster team unity. Be aware that residents are anxious to get back to their clinical responsibilities (e.g., working up new patients, handling discharges); one feature of hospital work is that patient care issues are always lurking in the background and sometimes even more urgently inserting themselves into the foreground to the point at which teaching has to be interrupted.

Teaching and Supervisory Opportunities in Hospital Psychiatry

> Thought flows in terms of stories—stories about events, stories about people, and stories about intentions and achievements.
> The best teachers are the best story tellers.
> We learn in the form of stories.
>
> *Frank Smith*

Lectures and Group Sessions

When time permits, many attendings like to hold small, informal teaching sessions with the residents and students who are on their team. This allows a seminar-like atmosphere and may give the attending a chance to go into depth in some area in which they have special interest or expertise. At the more formal level, those who are associated with a teaching program will have the opportunity to give lectures as part of the core curriculum for the medical students or residents. If you are actively involved in consultation work, you may wish to develop some lectures in that subspecialty, such as evaluation of capacity, assessment and management of delirium on the medical and surgical units, medical mimics of anxiety and depression, or somatoform illnesses. Those who favor inpatient work should be able to lecture on topics such as acute psychosis, assessment and treatment options for treatment-resistant depression, and inpatient management of border-line personality disorder patients. If your primary specialty is emergency psychiatry, you need to be well versed in acute evaluation and management of patients; suggestions for your PowerPoint topics would include differential diagnosis of psychosis, acute management of suicidal and violent patients in the psychiatric emergency department, and medical clearance for psychiatric admission. One nice spin-off effect of preparing these lectures, of course, is a chance to review the literature and to refine your own knowledge base.

Individual Supervision

Individual supervision probably will be used more with residents, but if you can free a few moments, one-on-one time spent with medical students reviewing a note in detail or critiquing an interview in real time will mark you as an extraordinary attending to them. Resident supervision in the hospital setting has a vastly different quality compared with outpatient psychiatric supervision in a clinic setting, which is usually much more structured and where scheduled supervisory sessions are the norm. Although you might wish to try to schedule some regular times with your residents in the hospital setting, hospital supervision may be more extemporaneous because of the unpredictability of the work, and supervisory time is often linked to review of new cases as they occur. However, within this framework, there is still room for good, old-fashioned review of difficult cases; exploration of the resident's approach; and strategizing together. Senior clinicians are familiar with training in which a supervisor points out a learner's blind spots and how this countertransference interferes with treatment. Is there a place for this kind of supervision? A more tactful way to approach this kind of situation today is just to highlight the clinical phenomenon: "I think there is a big component of personality pathology with this patient that is undermining your best efforts. What do you think of that idea?" A relational approach in which you share your own past difficulties with a similar patient from your own training can be particularly useful here. As the quote at the beginning of this section by Frank Smith highlights, and as cognitive psychologists have pointed out as well, we all learn best through pattern recognition rather than through lists of facts or symptoms. By the time you are a supervisor, you should have accumulated several favorite stories you can use to illustrate certain concepts and clinical dilemmas. These anecdotes also serve to humanize you to your trainees, especially if they show you in a position of uncertainty or bewilderment from which you had to find your way. And relatedly, when you and your learner see a remarkable clinical situation or a memorable reversal from the expected (a manic patient who no one thought would improve but did, a borderline patient who developed remarkable insight into his or her cutting behavior, a psychotic patient who actually had a rare encephalopathy), encourage your student to highlight and categorize the experience somehow, adding that patient to his or her memory bank for future use, and thus encouraging the learner to build up his or her own internal catalogue of prototypical presentations; sometimes, I might even say something like, "Keep this patient in your mind as the Platonic ideal of Capgras syndrome."

Starting Off a Rotation With a Resident or Student

A useful habit to develop as an attending is to sit down with your new residents individually at the beginning of the rotation and explore what they want to work on during your time together, whether it be psychopharmacology, psychiatric diagnosis, overall patient management, supportive therapy, interviewing technique, or some other area of interest. I have found it useful to ask, "What do you think your strong points are so far (from internship or other residency experiences)? And what are some areas that you want to improve?" And do not neglect teaching as a skill a resident may want to focus on, because a good training program will be turning out future clinicians and teachers. If this is a focus of interest, you should pay extra attention to guiding residents in their interactions with earlier-year residents and medical students and in modeling traits of curiosity, encouragement, and a scholarly approach to clinical work (e.g., directing medical students to look up articles pertinent to their patients). Periodically checking in with your residents as to their perception of their progress in their goals for themselves and how that matches with your view of their development will ensure that your final evaluation is not a surprise.

Medical students also should have some sort of orientation in which the goals and objectives of a psychiatric rotation are laid out in some detail. This is often not the province of a busy attending, but when it is done elsewhere (by a medical education director, for instance), your own briefer introduction incorporating specific goals for the students can be a good initiation to the work they will be doing.

Directive Teaching Versus Collaborative Teaching

> When mother-cow is chewing grass
> its young ones watch its mouth.
>
> *Chinua Achebe, Things Fall Apart*

> Teaching and learning are one shared endeavor, and great teachers
> inspire learners through a mutually interactive process that informs
> and creates community.
>
> *Laura Weiss Roberts*

Most of us are familiar with the so-called apprentice model of medical education in which a trainee, be it a resident or student, is essentially seen as an "empty vessel" to be filled with the attending's accumulated knowledge and wisdom. This model is associated with the directive teaching modalities that are so tempting to resort to when time is short. Speaking for myself, I would add that impatience or fatigue may cause an attending to favor this modality over the collaborative style I elaborate on shortly. Examples of this directive style of teaching include demonstrating how to do an interview while the learners observe, lecturing about an illness or a strategy of treatment, and intervening by interrupting a trainee's interaction with a patient and taking over an interview that is deemed to be off-track or going poorly. Modeling is an important element of teaching and supervision and can provide a modicum of comfort for the trainee at times. Students and residents do indeed want, as the Achebe quote says, to "see how we chew." They are interested in how experienced attendings relate to various patients, puzzle through a differential diagnosis, and interact with the treatment team. You can certainly build some "street cred" if you can do these things well and are an exemplar of solid clinical care. At the same time, it is easy to see how the sole use of this hierarchical model can leave learners feeling bored, disengaged, or even frankly undermined at times. Your trainees will retain knowledge better if they are more actively involved. To that end, you should strive to create the collaborative learning community Laura Roberts promotes in her quote at the beginning of this section, one in which residents and students, depending on their relative training level, have a degree of autonomy and are seen as capable of making their own valuable contributions to patient care. More advanced residents in particular will appreciate the opportunity to form clinical judgments and decisions themselves, knowing that you are available to tweak, amend, or just offer your imprimatur. Because I know that many of my residents want to moonlight at local community psychiatric hospitals on weekends before finishing their residency, one of my goals is to prepare them for that independent role through their hospital rotations. Watching me do interviews or prescribe medication combinations is not going to prepare them adequately!

A good example of a learner-centered approach to supervision is to observe a resident or student who is interviewing a patient, followed by soliciting their thoughts about the process, their reasoning about the differential diagnosis, and their ideas of how they might structure or layer a further clarifying workup of the patient. Many supervisors will use Socratic-type questions to guide the discussion, but the most important element is to show respect for the ideas proposed by the trainee, even while nudging toward modifications or greater depth of understanding. Help the trainees to develop an evidence-based approach to their treatment plan if they do not have the necessary knowledge base already. This might involve directing them toward certain readings such as case reports, review articles, or treatment guidelines.

Overall, you will ultimately find that residents and students respond to your enthusiasm and support more than pure scholarship and knowledge. Although some probing questions to lead a learner toward a wider differential can be useful, the days of "pimping" residents and students in a humiliating fashion are fortunately pretty much behind us (I recall one notorious internal medicine attending from my era whose interns needed β-blockers prior to his rounds!). Over time, I have come to favor the more open, reciprocal, collaborative, and interdependent teaching relationship that can coexist alongside the traditional "apprenticeship" model of medical education. The newer model is more in keeping with the current generation's expectations and is tailor-made for psychiatry because we already value the team approach and the input of all disciplines.

To further clarify, we also might say that this continuum from modeling to "watching with encouragement of reflection" should be congruent with the level of the learner, not just from medical student to senior resident but with your realistic assessment of where the particular learner is on his or her trajectory toward mastery of a particular skill, be it interviewing a psychotic patient, assessing a patient's risk factors and protective factors for self-harm, or informing a family of their young adult child's probable schizophrenia or borderline personality disorder diagnosis. In the final analysis, in deciding what admixture of directive and collaborative supervisory techniques to use so that trainees gain competency in these and other clinical skills, each attending must also negotiate a balance that will fit with the particular hospital setting and with his or her particular personality and teaching strengths.

Dealing Specifically With Different Levels of Learners

Medical Students

What should medical students come away with from a hospital psychiatric rotation? What do they want from a rotation, and how do they best learn? Several years ago, I sat down with a few students and canvassed them precisely about these issues. I found that they want to be included and that they like to be helpful in the care of patients. They also enjoy the format of conducting an uninterrupted interview with a patient with an immediate critique and discussion afterward. I tell my students that by the end of the rotation, I want them to be able to conduct a decent templated initial interview and subsequent interview for a progress note. When the occasional student gets ahead of himself or herself with an unfocused, meandering interview with the pretext of some semitherapeutic elements, my musical analogy has been the need to learn to play scales before embarking on sonatas.

Tell your team not to indulge in "swarm interviewing" during rounds (random firing of questions willy nilly at the patient rather than sequential progression of interviewing from medical student to resident to attending). This more systematic approach will allow the student to see how the resident and attending layer their interview questions and to see more clearly the nuanced interview techniques the residents and attending may use. By rotation's end, through their interviewing experiences, medical students should be able to perform a comprehensive suicide risk assessment, a review of depressive and psychotic symptoms, and a solid mental status examination. Medical student supervision and teaching also should be directed at their learning how to intersperse empathetic comments into their interactions and how to use basic principles of motivational interviewing.

Residents

One issue that may arise for the early career psychiatrist is that there may not be much of an age disparity between a young attending and his or her residents. At the simplest level lies the question of how they address you, but behind this appellation decision may lurk anxieties about your authority, competence, and perhaps even gender. Nonetheless, it is important to recognize that you do indeed know quite a lot more than the second-year residents with whom you will be mostly working, and you likely have much to offer even to very senior residents. One advantage of being a young attending is that residents will be able to relate to you easily; the danger is that an overidentification with your generational cohort could interfere with supervision and teaching and stifle honest critique when necessary. All things considered, what I have observed from my senior vantage point of young attending colleagues with their residents is a friendly generational comfort that fosters a collaborative approach to patient care.

As you get to know your residents with their strengths and areas of challenge, try to determine what kind of learners they are and what is the best way to approach each of them. Do they learn best from articles, hearing the information spoken, diagrams, modeling, or just a few brief comments after your observation? Identify your residents' cognitive style and emotive style and help them see where it will be effective or not without psychoanalyzing them. Some residents are very medical model oriented and already fairly skilled with diagnosis, medications, and time management. Others have a natural flare for the relationship part of the interaction with the patient. Each group will have to strengthen the component of care they are less adept at but also should be encouraged to retain and even build on the areas of natural talent or predilection. Try to identify this early on in your meetings with the residents and with your initial observations of their patient interactions.

Although it is time-consuming, I personally like to review and edit resident notes. I see this as part of supervision because it gives me a chance to see how the resident is cognitively structuring the day-to-day progress of the patient. In addition, I have come to recognize that not all residents have acquired writing skills commensurate with their knowledge base. In fact, this issue is important not only for quality hospital documentation but also because your supervision mission should include alertness to opportunities for scholarly projects, prime examples of which are posters for conferences and case reports for journals. Encouraging residents to get involved in such activities and supervising their work or coauthoring can be a nice supplement to everyday teaching. Our residents have used patient material from the hospital setting for presenting posters at American Psychiatric Association and Association for Academic Psychiatry annual meetings, for instance. Some residents have even presented workshops based on their inpatient experiences.

Supportive Psychotherapy as Psychological Training

Residents are fascinated by the psychological aspect of a hospital patient's presentation but are not confident in their assessment of this aspect of the interview, which is usually the weakest part of their formulation. Most psychiatric residencies are organized so that hospital experiences precede outpatient clinic assignments and training in psychotherapy. This was indeed true for me years ago and is the case with our residents today. This means that residents rely mostly on their common sense, the quality of their own upbringing, and whatever counseling or quasi-counseling roles they have had (e.g., resident assistant in a college dorm, youth groups, suicide hotline volunteer) in being therapeutic with their patients. The concept of supportive psychotherapy, which is considered a core graduation competency for psychiatry residents, is actually a comfortable modality at all levels of training and can be a good stopgap in the early years of training and in the hospital services. The ability to know when to offer various elements of support (e.g., advice, encouragement, clarification, reality testing) is almost intuitive to many learners but can be further refined with some guidance. I have found that just "naming" the supportive technique the resident was using, often unaware, is beneficial: "That was a good example of clarification." So try to provide some basic tools of supportive therapy—even those from your own knowledge of cognitive-behavioral therapy, dialectical behavior therapy, motivational interviewing, or basic psychodynamics—in your supervision and teaching with early-year residents. This will be especially important for their work with patients who are not flagrantly psychotic, manic, depressed to the point of needing electroconvulsive therapy, and the like. Many patients present to the psychiatric emergency department or inpatient unit or are on medical units requesting psychiatric input but are in a psychologically based crisis state, and medication will not be the primary mode of treatment. Young patients coming into a psychiatric emergency department or even subsequently admitted short-term for depressive reactions caused by some stressor, such as a romantic breakup, are good candidates for supportive interventions. In fact, patients recovering from a psychotic state who are now debating whether they are willing to take medications as an outpatient may benefit from supportive techniques that address denial. Once a patient begins to have some degree of reality testing, I usually encourage my team to try to destigmatize psychosis with a little pep talk to the patient saying something like this: "You know, John, under the right circumstances, anybody can start to see things or hear things, like if they had a high fever or someone put something in their drink. Your brain just did it on its own, that's all." If your residents do not have ways of thinking about these cases other than pharmacologically, they will feel adrift.

Residents as "Junior Attendings"

At the most advanced end of the teaching continuum are those senior residents who are about to graduate and may wish to spend some time as a "junior attending" on a hospital psychiatric service before embarking on their careers. You as the attending have the very gratifying opportunity to apply the final layer of polish to their training; you will be watching closely and providing feedback to them as they run the team meetings; teach the earlier-year residents and students; and interact with social workers, nurses, and other staff. Here is your chance to be "teaching about teaching," passing on to the next generation the useful didactic approaches and various pearls that are not codified in manuals or guidelines.

Keep in mind that another corollary function of a teacher and supervisor is that of a mentor. At the resident level, trainees solicit advice not only about clinical judgment and techniques but also about professional development and career trajectory. Some of my most recent examples include questions such as: "Should I do a fellowship or go straight into practice after my fourth year?"; "What electives should I consider in my fourth year?"; and "What are the pros and cons of private practice versus academia?" Of course, these kinds of questions are rather easy to discuss, and if you are a young attending, all the better, as you will have had more immediate experience with these crossroad points. But residents may bring you thornier problems as well: trouble with a particular supervisor, conflict with a nurse, or personal issues interfering with patient care. Sometimes your advice and support will suffice, but be careful not to overstep your role and know when you need to enlist or recommend additional avenues for assistance (the residency director, for instance).

The "Borderline Talk"

Every trainee must learn the skill of a frank discussion about a patient's unique issues. Whether this involves substance use, maladaptive relationships, or the new onset of a long-term disorder, this skill can be taught and learned. One example of such a skill is the disclosure of the diagnosis to a patient with borderline personality disorder. The ability to elucidate to a patient and family what the lifelong history of mood instability represents diagnostically is a skill that every resident should acquire during training. This means that you as a supervisor should have perfected a "spiel" to tell your residents in certain situations when bipolarity has been ruled out. You can develop your own particular spin, but a good borderline talk should include some common elements, including the clinical features of borderline personality disorder, the possible genetic and biological components (lessens some of the guilt and blame), the treatability with good therapies, and the futility of trying medication after medication. Let your residents try a few of these frank conversations with select patients during the rotation. Prepare them that a certain percentage of patients will remain wedded to their mood disorder diagnoses and their polypharmacy cocktails, but the patient's negative reaction will at least allow the resident to practice some supportive probing, such as "What do you not like about the borderline personality disorder diagnosis?"

Vignette

A 19-year-old female student was admitted from the medical unit after treatment for an intentional overdose. She seemingly reconstituted quickly, and there was pressure from her family for her to get back to school so she wouldn't get "off-track." Something did not quite seem "real" about her recovery. The resident was encouraged to explore further with her and uncovered previously undisclosed borderline features with ongoing suicidal fantasies and wishes that would put her at risk outside the hospital. The supervision thus was directed at not accepting the pressure from the family, the insurance provider, and the patient for a premature discharge. The resident then worked in a supportive fashion on safety planning and distress tolerance until the patient truly stabilized and discharge to outpatient became a safer option.

Vignette

A 20-year-old male college student was admitted in a manic state. He responded well to medication in the hospital after a tumultuous course requiring intensive nursing monitoring and a several-week stay. Once stabilized, he wanted to return immediately to his very difficult engineering course load, even though we believed that his cognitive ability had not totally returned to normal and that a full course load so soon could set him up for failure (and even a relapse). The general teaching point involved was that the resident and student could use their relationship to the patient and their knowledge of the stress of university coursework to offer supportive advice to him about the need to temporarily cut back on his credit hours.

This case could be adapted for several teaching purposes. The medical student was enlisted to meet one-on-one with the patient to discuss his credit load and even the possibility of a semester off from school; this is actually a form of supportive psychotherapy, and articles were given to the student on that topic (the concept of advice as temporarily "lending your ego" to a person under distress). The resident concentrated more on the pharmacology of mania treatment, adjusting the blood levels of the mood stabilizer, and the phenomenology of manic illness. He spent time reviewing these concepts with the students and took the lead in using the Young Mania Rating Scale with consensus ratings among the team members after interviews.

All of this supervised clinical care—the medical student doing supportive therapy, use of a consensus rating of mania during rounds, supervision of the resident's teaching—did not happen spontaneously or magically but rather was set up for them as an experience. For a lot of students, this degree of involvement is what will make the psychiatry rotation memorable; for residents, the degree and variety of responsibility under supervision will round them out as more complete hospital psychiatrists and encourage clinician or educator roles in the future.

Final Thoughts for Teachers
Find Your Niche but Do Not Be Monolithic

Every psychiatrist, especially in an academic setting, will have areas of interest and concentration, specializations, even pet peeves, *idées fixes*, and diagnostic predilections. Like it or not, you may end up "typecast," but hopefully it will be in a role that suits you and is useful in the overall education of trainees at your institution. You can influence this to some extent. In our department, for instance, we have a whole range of experts in different areas, not always by design. One colleague is known for the skillful "borderline talk" he gives to patients who have been misguided by multiple previous treating clinicians into thinking that they have bipolar disorder; another colleague is a master of the catatonia examination. Because my training was in the Jurassic period, I am saddled with the reputation of being a psychiatrist who considers—and teaches—psychological and psychodynamic factors in the hospital setting. In fact, one time one of my colleagues said, "This patient has a lot of psychodynamics—it would be a good case for Dr. Casher!" Desired or imposed, whatever teaching niche you end up occupying, if you want to be a top-notch hospital teacher of residents and students, make sure you also retain a solid base as an all-around diagnostician and psychopharmacologist and have familiarity with various therapies.

Vignette

When I was interviewing for psychiatry residencies years ago, one California program had Erik Erikson on the faculty! "Wow," I said to the senior resident interviewing me, "you're so lucky!" (I had read *Childhood and Society* in college and knew Erikson was a link to Freud himself.) The resident surprised and disillusioned me [Is that why I remember it so clearly now?] with his reply: "Stages of man, stages of man! If I have to hear that phrase one more time, I think I'll go crazy!"

Moral of the story: Don't become too enamored of your own ideas. Don't become a broken record. Don't become a parody of yourself.

Teaching Is a Generative Endeavor

When you look at effective teachers in any field, one quality they have is an ability to move beyond a focus on themselves and to actively engage the learner, often communicating or eliciting an emotional response alongside the concepts or techniques being taught or demonstrated. In Erik Erikson's Stages of Psychosocial Development, we would say that they have successfully navigated the stage of Generativity versus Stagnation (at least in this arena)—that is, they are shepherding in, for example, the next generation of physicians and psychiatrists. The students, on the contrary, are hopefully possessed of a solid fundamental identity in classic Eriksonian terms—that should have been settled in late adolescence—but at a higher transformative level, they are forming their "professional identities," and poor supervision and teaching in an unstructured program will hamper their successful traversal of this career developmental stage. What does this mean at the more mundane level? For me, it means I revel in seeing my students and residents do well: be able to bring down a difficult manic patient, stop me in the hallway to tell me they matched at their first choice for internal medicine (which they interviewed at during their psychiatry rotation), convince a patient with borderline personality disorder that she can forgo that cocktail of medications because she doesn't have bipolar disorder after all, write their first journal article, or even join our faculty when they graduate.

The renowned psychiatrist Glen Gabbard, M.D., makes another point about teaching that is good to keep in mind. He reminds us that teaching means that you are "always learning." Teaching forces you to clarify your thoughts, to explain yourself, to keep up with the literature as much as you can, and to be open to new ideas from the next generations.

KEY POINTS

- The psychiatric hospital services, with their wide range of acute patients, offer great opportunities to teach psychiatry.

- Although the hospital sections (consultation-liaison, inpatient, psychiatric emergency department) have commonalities, each also has specific areas to master that provide teaching and supervisory opportunities.

- Learn to adjust your teaching not only to the level of trainees but also to their particular strengths and weaknesses and to their various learning styles.

- Collaborative learning approaches that are less hierarchical and value the input of the trainee will engage your learners to a greater degree and are more in keeping with generational expectations.

- Teaching can have positive effects on you by keeping you engaged and up-to-date in the field and generative toward the upcoming young physicians and can become one of your most gratifying professional activities.

PART III
Clinical Care

CHAPTER 8

Initial Assessment and Treatment Planning

Heather E. Schultz, M.D., M.P.H.

Initial Assessment

As a hospital psychiatrist, you will meet patients for the first time in a variety of settings—from the psychiatric emergency department to the inpatient unit to the medical floor. In each of these areas, your initial contact should achieve several crucial aims:

- *To perform an assessment of patients' current presentation, with a focus on what brought them into the hospital acutely*—Narrow in on details about their current mental health symptoms, psychiatric history, and treatment including therapy and medications. Gain an understanding of their psychosocial stressors and an estimation of their ability to engage coping skills when in crisis.
- *To assess acute safety, especially in emergency and consult settings*—Asking patients about their thoughts of harming themselves and others and obtaining collateral information about their acute safety often determine the level of supervision needed. For instance, you may need to dictate

whether a patient may be discharged home, needs one-on-one supervision, or needs security on standby when evaluated because of agitation.

- *To review patients' medical history and generally assess their overall health*—Numerous medical conditions present with psychiatric symptoms—from dementia to thyroid disease to medication side effects.
- *To decipher what patients' objectives are and whether they are willing to be involved in treatment*—Clarifying their goals can reduce interpersonal friction and enhance the psychiatrist-patient alliance.
- *To develop a differential diagnosis in line with the patient's presenting symptoms*—At times, this is broad because the case is complex or information is missing.
- *To determine treatment options that are likely to help the patient*—Treatment options range from medications to electroconvulsive therapy (ECT) to substance abuse treatment.
- *To communicate a plan with the rest of the team from nursing staff to consultants*—Nothing is more disquieting than discovering that a patient at high risk for harm to self or others has been allowed to leave the hospital against medical advice.
- To consider steps that must be taken before a safe discharge

First Impressions Matter

Meeting a patient in the hospital setting for the first time comes with some challenges. Some patients may request to speak with a psychiatrist because of concerns about their emotional well-being, whereas others may view you as the grim reaper coming with news of their impending doom (with fears of hospitalization or a diagnosis of "crazy"). Despite persistent and rampant stigma about mental health issues, some patients are more seasoned in receiving psychiatric treatment. For instance, some individuals have had depression for decades and have had numerous medication trials and other treatment approaches, such as transcranial magnetic stimulation or ECT. These patients may know their history well and have strong opinions about which medications work and which do not. Alternatively, they may feel completely hopeless about potential recovery and convinced that their symptoms cannot be treated at all. Understanding patients' perspective on whether they need to see a psychiatrist, if medications or therapy may be useful, and previous treatment outcomes can generate important information up front that will aid rapport building and inform your approach to treatment. Furthermore, approaching patients with some flexibility and adjusting to their tone (which may range from eager to suspicious to dismissive) can smooth out the interpersonal kinks that may happen as a result of patients' own perceptions of their need for mental health treatment or lack thereof.

What to Know
Before the Patient Encounter

Before meeting with a patient for the first time, it is prudent to review the available medical records. In addition to past psychiatric outpatient visits and hospitalizations, review notes from visits with the primary care physician and to the emergency department. You may find information about recent medication changes or even changes in mood or behavior. If your electronic medical record links to outside hospital records, sort through those for any recent interactions with psychiatry (while maintaining Health Insurance Portability and Accountability Act [HIPAA] compliance, because some records may need the patient's permission before being released). This can provide important background information that will lead your assessment in the right direction. Having a recent medication list in hand will save you time if a patient has forgotten a medication name or if the conversation is emotionally laden. Also, some detective work comes in handy when a patient reports never having seen a psychiatrist, but you discover numerous past psychiatric hospitalizations and medication trials! Being kind with the background information you gain is essential, because patients may feel embarrassed or guarded about their history or are experiencing mania, psychosis, or dementia and simply may not remember it.

Help Trainees With the
Structure and Goals of the Interview

When working as a team with trainees, knowing both *who* is going to ask the patient questions and *what* they need to ask is crucial to a smooth patient encounter. Often, a medical student will start the patient interview. Your coaching in advance to prepare the medical students to introduce themselves and their role and the reason for the interview will provide the framework for the initial assessment. Instead of reiterating what was read in the chart, the student may open the conversation by saying something like the following:

> Hello Mr. X, I'm Brendan, and I'm a third-year medical student rotating with the psychiatry consult team. Your primary team was concerned that you might be experiencing some trouble with your mood, so we are here to ask you more about that. I did have a chance to review your chart and saw that you have a listed diagnosis of major depressive disorder. Can you tell me how your moods have been recently?

Teaching medical students to provide the context of who they are and why they may ask potentially sensitive questions and to frame the interview as an introduction can prevent errors in communication. Patients may ask, "How much would you like to know?" or "Should I start from the beginning?" It prevents mutual frustration to answer with parameters to guide conversation, such as "I would like to know how you have been feeling for the past 2 weeks." Coach the student to use open-ended questions, to keep the interview conversational, and to avoid prematurely giving a diagnosis or medical advice until the team has discussed the case. Prepare a strategy for times when the medical student might run out of questions to ask or the patient becomes impatient or irritable. A resident physician then may ask further clarifying questions and fill in any gaps in the patient's history, followed by a few final questions by the attending. If an area needs to be further explored, avoid asking the same questions again but instead reiterate what you know and ask for clarification. For instance, "I understand that you've been depressed for many years with suicidal thoughts in the past. When you took extra trazodone a few nights ago, were you having suicidal thoughts?" Avoid talking over other members of the team or interrupting them. Sometimes, patients are reluctant to speak with trainees, but often words of support from the attending such as "This medical student has been working hard on the team and is invested in your care" can put the patient at ease. In the case of a patient who is a medical student or physician, it may be wise to limit a team interaction with him or her if he or she is sensitive about privacy issues (for instance, he or she lectures at a teaching hospital), but defer to the patient's wishes.

Use Your Knowledge of DSM to Guide Questions

A good medical assessment begins with open-ended questions that allow patients to tell their stories. However, at a certain point, there may need to be clarification of symptoms to distinguish between disorders. For example, imagine the patient who presents with this story:

> You see Doc, I've been struggling with mood swings for as long as I can remember, but I have been feeling really Jekyll and Hyde lately. One minute I can be really happy, and the next I'm causing a scene and breaking up with my boyfriend for the twentieth time that day. I've been diagnosed with bipolar disorder in the past, but medications haven't helped much. Then again, I never take them for long. My sleep depends on how excited I am about life.

Based on this history alone, the interviewer should consider the possibility of a bipolar mood disorder versus borderline personality disorder.

Further questioning about the frequency and duration of mood swings, number of sleep hours per night, level of impulsivity, history of psychosis, interpersonal sensitivity, and so forth should clarify the diagnosis. Your familiarity with DSM, or at the very least having it available to compare symptoms with criteria, will allow the information provided by a patient to fit an accurate differential diagnosis. In addition, a thorough history may identify important data points to be considered even when the initial diagnosis appears obvious. For instance, a patient could present with symptoms of paranoia, auditory hallucinations, and disorganized behavior. Although a thought disorder such as schizophrenia is possible, questions about substance use could determine that symptoms occur only in the context of intoxication. The essence of clinical skill is to find and recognize patterns that lead to an accurate diagnosis, but to have all the facts is the first essential.

Talk About Discharge During Your First Meeting

Whether it be in the psychiatric emergency department, in the hospital on the consult service, or on an inpatient unit, patients often want to know when they can go home. For those with tumultuous family relationships, intolerable roommates, or homelessness, staying in the hospital may provide a needed escape from stressors. Psychotic patients may become paranoid, believe that there is a conspiracy against them, and perceive that the hospital is not a safe place. Alternatively, patients may minimize psychiatric symptoms because they want to return home. Whatever the case may be, it is important to ask the patient how he or she feels about being in the hospital when you first meet him or her. Answers can vary from "I feel I will need to stay here for a long time" to "This has all been a terrible miscommunication, and I need to leave." Set expectations regarding the criteria a patient should meet before discharge. For instance, you could tell a patient "I would like to work with you to make sure your mood is stable, your thoughts are clear, and you are not at risk for harming yourself or others." Concurrently, get collateral information from outpatient providers, family, and others to help you judge the patient's level of risk and readiness for discharge. If it seems as though a patient may be difficult to discharge because of dependent traits, attachment to the sick role, or avoidance of real world stressors, be sure to explain the limitations of treatment in the hospital and the goals for outpatient care. Choose a potential date for discharge and focus on safety planning as effective ways to set mutual expectations for both the psychiatrist and the patient, even in an initial meeting.

Divide or Delegate Work

It does not make sense for everyone to contact the patient's family, outpatient psychiatrist, and therapist. Just as a patient does not want to repeat the story numerous times, sources of collateral information also may become frustrated with numerous conversations with members of the health care team. Thus, a plan for communication among the team and time to compare notes in person, in addition to documenting these conversations in the medical record, is essential. In the psychiatric emergency setting, it may even be practical for you to interview a child or adolescent patient while the social worker speaks with the parents. This expedites the evaluation and may allow each person interviewed to be more open with their stories than they would be if interviewed together. In the inpatient setting, the social worker may speak with the therapist while you call the outpatient physician. Documentation of these conversations provides a more thorough assessment of the patient and often guides relevant treatment decisions. For instance, an outpatient psychiatrist may say, "I've wanted to recommend a medication washout period with consideration for an MAOI but did not feel this was safe to start outside of the hospital." This can then become a collaborative treatment approach, and the initial changes to medications can be more smoothly continued when the patient returns to the outpatient team.

Treatment Planning

To Medicate or Not to Medicate

Once a differential diagnosis is established, the next step is to think about possible interventions. Although the question "Does this patient need medication for these psychiatric symptoms?" seems simple and intuitive, coming to the answer can prove to be challenging. Many patients in the hospital are presenting in the midst of a psychosocial crisis, such as a breakup or divorce, loss of a job, or impending homelessness. Psychological stressors may prove less tangible; does a person feel as though current academic stress equates to him or her internalizing failure as an identity? Has a patient suppressed emotional reactions from trauma and instead taken a deep dive into the underworld of substance abuse or self-harm? Understanding the patient's psychiatric history as well as the chief complaint for the current hospital encounter often will allow you to theorize how much a medication option could be helpful. For some patients, the answer is clear. If you have ever spent time in a room with someone who is acutely manic, with pressured speech, wild hand gestures, and grand plans to take over the world, no amount of discussion can resolve this presentation. The choice of a medication such as an antipsychotic, mood stabilizer, or benzodiazepine may depend on the patient's history with medications, such as previous trials and whether he or she has a history of alcohol abuse or other illicit substance use. On the contrary, an anxiously avoidant patient who cannot confront the boss about an increasingly overwhelming workload may have significant relief once able to advocate and problem solve appropriately. Supportive therapy without medications may be enough to help in this situation. We often see medications as tools. For instance, a patient who presents with new-onset psychotic symptoms in the context of excessive marijuana use would likely benefit from an antipsychotic, and yet time will tell if the psychosis persists outside of substance use. Delirious patients may need the same antipsychotic because they are so uncomfortably confused that every minute becomes disorienting and distressing, but once their medical issue has resolved, their presentation returns to their previous baselines. Thus, medication might be used here as a short-term solution until diagnostic clarity over time has been achieved.

Psychotherapy

Some patients may prefer to focus on a therapeutic approach to treatment and to defer medications because of apprehension or a history of side effects. Consider whether medications are essential and if any therapy modalities may prove effective. For instance, if you are consulted to discuss a patient's grief reaction to a new diagnosis of cancer, it might not be wise to jump to a diagnosis of major depression until the timeline and symptoms are clear. In this case, supportive therapy may go a long way with a patient who is suffering. There are creative ways to provide patients with additional layers of support, such as working with a psychologist, spiritual care worker, or social work staff. A cohesive team can strategize about how to use therapy to intervene acutely and then to consider appropriate outpatient follow-up options. Interestingly, there can be too much therapy in the acute setting. Take, for instance, the patient with an extensive trauma history. To unpack traumatic memories with that patient may lead to retraumatization, regression, or worsening mood symptoms. Consider the time limitations of hospitalization and remember that, ultimately, a good treatment plan includes discharge. To tell patients that they may share anything with you and then to send them home within a few days can come across as invalidating, so set limits and a framework around the goals that you can work on in the acute setting. Teach coping skills to use in times of distress via a dialectical behavior model, because these skills can translate to the outpatient environment and become a part of the patient's safety plan.

Collaborate With the Patient

In the mid-twentieth century, physicians typically did not share medical diagnoses with patients. This separation of experts in a paternalistic and omniscient culture from patients, who even today can be viewed more as their diagnosis than as whole persons, creates a conflict. If, for instance, a patient is highly manic, to share your opinion about that state of mind may be met with arguments, agitation, or dismissal. However, if you do not share your thoughts with a patient at all, it may erode the potential for a trusting therapeutic relationship. Attempt to establish a rapport with your patient by understanding his or her goals for hospitalization (or the wish to leave). Being able to reflect on what is important to the patient, such as a return to work or hobbies, will create a foundation for a discussion about discharge plans.

The Difficult Patient

For a variety of reasons, it is difficult to care for some patients. It is natural to feel frightened of an agitated patient who has a history of assaulting physicians or angry at a patient who has offensive beliefs. However, essential qualities of a psychiatrist include professionalism and compassion. Discuss countertransference reactions with the rest of the team to create a sense of accountability. Furthermore, it reminds us that we are all human and that sometimes we will feel unexpected or uncomfortable reactions when faced with a patient who triggers an emotional response. It is important for us to hold ourselves accountable for those feelings, regardless of how challenging or provocative a patient is, and to maintain a professional rapport with the best intentions for the patient in mind. Be careful to make treatment decisions with the patient's best interests in mind, even when interactions become emotionally charged or challenging.

Where Will the Patient Go When Leaving the Hospital?

Once patients are stable enough to leave the acute setting, it is vital to consider a smooth transition to outpatient care so that their acute safety or mental health treatment is not disrupted. Potential discharge options are numerous, and each requires a different set of considerations.

Return Home

Returning home is the most common discharge after a patient is psychiatrically evaluated in the hospital setting. If patients are not an acute danger to themselves or others and able to care for themselves, they typically will be discharged home with a safety plan. This entails that they can identify warning signs that they are decompensating and have coping skills to use when distressed, people to reach out to for support, and mechanisms to ensure that the environment is safe (for instance, removing firearms).

Discharge to Family or Friends

Patients may need extra support when discharged from the hospital because of safety risks (e.g., someone who has long-standing suicidal thoughts) or the need for help with daily life. For example, a college student who has experienced major depressive symptoms may have a parent come to provide support after discharge. Or an older patient who has some difficulties with daily tasks such as cooking and cleaning may decide with family that it is best not to live alone.

Homelessness

Unfortunately, many patients with chronic mental illness also have persistent problems with secure housing because of difficulties with employment, comorbid substance abuse, or even paranoia about their living situation. To connect with their outpatient team, such as community mental health, about possible shelters, programs, and assistance can be useful in safety planning.

Partial Hospitalization Program

Partial hospitalization has become a more accessible option as these programs become more common. For many patients, a bridge between an inpatient hospitalization and returning to work or school can be helpful to strengthen their coping skills through therapy programming. Most of these programs meet for the day, and patients return home at night unless their acute safety is jeopardized.

Adult Foster Care

Patients who may not be able to fully care for their activities of daily living because of chronic mental illness may require an adult foster care home for support, with staff members to assist with paying bills, acquiring meals, and providing medications on a schedule. Placement may require coordination with a guardian because this setting is often a good fit for patients who lack insight into their need for mental health treatment but who can be stabilized on medication.

Subacute Rehabilitation Program

Some patients who are physically debilitated may need to do more physical therapy or have skilled nursing needs. This plan is often initiated by physical and occupational therapists, who can recommend an appropriate level of care and coordinate with care managers to arrange this care.

Outpatient Substance Use Treatment

Patients with substance use disorders may seek resources in the community such as Alcoholics Anonymous and see a psychiatrist who specializes in addiction.

Inpatient Substance Use Treatment

Patients who have relapsed while in the outpatient substance use treatment setting, or who are in active withdrawal, may fear continued use if discharged home and need a higher level of care to address their addiction. An inpatient substance treatment setting is especially appropriate for patients who are motivated and insightful regarding their wish to pursue sobriety. Those who are precontemplative may struggle with the restrictions of this environment (treatment can last for weeks to months), and the risks and benefits of inpatient treatment versus relapse should be discussed candidly.

Residential Treatment

Although somewhat uncommon, residential treatment can be a useful longer-term treatment option for patients who have struggled to maintain stability outside of a structured setting. Patients who have eating disorders, personality disorders, or substance use may do well in this longer-term, more therapy-inclined approach to treatment. Often, patients are limited by finances, as these settings can be expensive and are not always covered by insurance.

State Hospital

State hospitals have become a less common placement option over time because many have shut down over the years. For the patient who is persistently and severely struggling with mental illness and is not able to be placed elsewhere safely or cared for by family, this is a long-term treatment option, but the wait lists for admission tend to be long.

Jail or Police Custody

When patients are brought into the hospital in police custody, often because they have been charged with a crime and their safety is also a concern, the decision about discharge back to police and possibly jail is an important one. Although it is nearly impossible to do a quick forensic evaluation in the acute setting, the patients' past diagnoses and current symptoms will help you differentiate antisocial personality traits and malingering from an acute disorder of thought or mood. Many jail settings have a mental health service, and often recommendations can be made to their treatment teams, ranging from medications to suicide precautions, before patients return to jail.

Contingency Plans

When a patient is admitted to the inpatient unit, there may be a long list of prescriptions or no medications at all. Although there might be admission order sets used by your health care system that include medications to be used on an "as-needed" basis for agitation, anxiety, or insomnia, it is vital to consider each patient's individual case when writing and reviewing admission orders. For instance, a patient with panic attacks or catatonia would likely benefit from an as-needed benzodiazepine order, but a patient with a history of polysubstance abuse or recent delirium would not. A good rule of thumb is that there is not a one-size-fits-all order set, and it is important to be thoughtful about what patients might need for anxiety, agitation, or pain. The idea of "chemical restraints" is dangerous and unethical and should be avoided. However, if a patient becomes unexpectedly agitated, it is important to have planned out an approach to maintain the safety of both patients and staff. For instance, if a manic patient becomes acutely agitated in the middle of the night because of racing thoughts or paranoid delusions, and a nurse is concerned about that patient attacking the staff, then it is likely appropriate to give the patient a medication for agitation, such as an antipsychotic. Nurses may use an algorithm to score agitation to document reasons for the need for these medications. Having these orders available as needed and in advance may prevent a delay in a time-sensitive situation of escalating agitation (see Chapter 11, "Acute Disorders").

Coordination of Care With Outpatient Providers

If a patient has been seen by an outpatient therapist or psychiatrist, then it is not only standard practice but also professional courtesy to connect with the patient's outpatient providers. This requires patient permission, and a release of information signed by the patient is ideal. However, in some emergency situations, a psychiatrist may seek collateral information from those who know a patient well without releasing information to them. This may be particularly relevant in the psychiatric emergency department where patients may present with acute suicidality, psychosis, mania, or altered mental status. To expedite a safe and thoughtful decision about treatment and disposition, knowing more about a patient's history is usually crucial.

Even if a patient has met with a psychiatrist only a handful of times, his or her first impressions and understanding of the patient's narrative can be diagnostically valuable. If the patient has a long-standing relationship with a therapist or psychiatrist, then he or she may be able to guide you regarding therapeutic approaches and medications that have either worked well or created trouble for the patient in the past. At times, there may be a difference of opinion between the hospital psychiatrist and the outpatient team about a patient's diagnosis or the optimal medications that should be used for treatment. Remember that patients can present differently when they are in distress and also that the luxury of observing the patient throughout the day in the hospital may add context to this difference in perspective. Inpatient and outpatient psychiatrists may be familiar with different medications based on their practice style, such as attention to cost, availability of medication samples, and preference for or against newer medications. Beware of splitting, as patients might complain about their outpatient team (or conversely, idealize them), and you should aim to create an alliance with both the patient and the outpatient providers. This creates a smooth transition for transferring care and prevents the urge to "rescue" the patient from suboptimal treatment, which could be the case but more often reflects a patient's frustration with his or her mental health issues. Sharing new information with the outpatient team also helps them moving forward—for instance, the patient with "rapid-cycling bipolar disorder" may in fact be having mood swings throughout the day and fit diagnostic criteria for borderline personality disorder. Describing this to the outpatient team could shift the treatment approach from medication focus to more therapy-intensive modalities, such as dialectical behavior therapy. Conversely, your diagnosis of a straightforward depression may have to be reconsidered when you learn from the outpatient caregiver about the patient's unacknowledged alcohol use disorder.

Adjust the Course as Needed

Even a seasoned psychiatrist may be met with unanticipated challenges during the course of treatment. Unexpected medication side effects or lack of effect, new acute stressors that affect a patient's mood, or collateral information that complicates discharge planning are all potential reasons to adjust treatment plans or even reconsider a discharge. It is important to be flexible and to lean on the observations of the interdisciplinary team during these times. Did a patient who you believed was receiving a therapeutic dose of a mood stabilizer stay up all night and then loudly sing during an art therapy group? To be able to take a step back and to reassess and recon-figure a treatment plan takes self-awareness, humility, and, most impor-tantly, an investment in observation of the patient. This may prevent the patient from being discharged home prematurely, especially if active safety issues are present. When adjusting a treatment plan, communicate clearly with both the team and the patient about your concerns, the proposed in-tervention (e.g., adding another medication), and a new anticipated dis-charge date. Many people can adapt to new information when they understand why it is happening, whereas they may feel trapped or misled without a relatively transparent discussion.

When in Doubt, Ask for Help

The final piece of advice that anyone working in a hospital setting can use almost universally is that it is always reasonable to consult with colleagues. In fact, this is a huge perk of working in an academic or a community set-ting. Discussion with a colleague when a case does not make sense, or when no apparent improvement is seen in the patient's symptoms, or when a dis-charge feels risky can add a helpful layer of perspective. Even if the consul-tation does not yield new information, it can provide you with reassurance that you have not overlooked or misinterpreted anything, allowing you to move forward with confidence.

Documentation

Finally, make sure that you document the rationale for your thought pro-cess when formulating your assessment and treatment plan. Clear medical records can assist future physicians in their understanding of a patient's psy-chiatric history and response to treatment. It will also be helpful in promot-ing continued insurance coverage of the patient's hospitalization. Finally, it reflects an assessment of risk in the case of an adverse event. Keep docu-mentation concise, nonjudgmental, and updated to ensure an accurate rep-resentation of the patient's course. (See Chapter 12, "Transitions in Care, Documentation, and Interdisciplinary Communication.")

KEY POINTS

- Your initial goals of assessment include understanding the patient's current and longitudinal history, safety risks, goals of treatment, dif-ferential diagnosis, and treatment options.

- Begin discharge planning with the first encounter as an integral part of hospital-based treatment.

- Medications and psychotherapies are tools to be used as indicated by the clinical situation; use them intentionally and judiciously.

- Consider the patient's likely postdischarge placement as you make hospital-based treatment decisions.

- Be flexible and open to input from patients, families, outpatient providers, and colleagues whom you consult.

CHAPTER 9

Diagnostic and Treatment Modalities

Joshua Bess, M.D.

The hospital setting not only lends itself to specific treatment modalities but also provides those treatments in ways that may differ from those in less acute settings. It is essential that you be familiar with each treatment, either to provide it personally or to incorporate it appropriately into a comprehensive therapeutic plan. In some cases, such as electroconvulsive therapy (ECT), hospital-based care may be used solely for the purpose of providing the treatment. In most instances, however, the acuity and severity of the pathology determine the level of care.

Numerous factors have contributed to the increased acuity of individuals admitted to inpatient psychiatry over the past few decades, primarily the expense of hospitalization and availability of outpatient services. Lengths of stay have decreased markedly for the same reasons. Patients are now admitted because of a crisis or an intensity of symptoms, not because they have a particular diagnosis. It is critical under these circumstances to make the most efficient use of the tools available in both the assessment and the treatment of your patients.

Diagnostic Testing

For many patients, this will be their first interaction with the mental health system for a first severe depressive episode, psychotic break, or another disorder. You and the inpatient psychiatry team must coordinate an appropriate diagnostic workup. In the short term, treatment focuses on alleviation of symptoms and suffering, but an accurate diagnosis is also essential to inform the plan for medium- or long-term treatment, establish prognosis, identify necessary psychosocial interventions and support, and justify payment for the hospital's services.

Medical Issues

Many psychiatric inpatients have limited access to general medical care or at least have not been evaluated within the several months—sometimes several years—leading to psychiatric admission. Although your comfort level practicing "regular medicine" will vary depending on your background, interest, and time in practice, your team is well placed to address nonpsychiatric problems as needed. Appropriate consultation with other hospital specialists and coordination with outpatient providers can contribute to helpful changes in current treatments or initiation of new treatment to manage acute and chronic medical problems. Especially be on the lookout for situations in which, because of the presenting complaint or the patient's psychiatric history, appropriate medical workup was not done because symptoms were attributed to "psychiatric issues."

Medications and other somatic therapies can alter physiology in important, often detrimental ways. Specific classes of medications (mostly notably, antipsychotics) may cause both short- and long-term medical problems, such as metabolic issues, requiring medical monitoring. Some medications, such as lithium, have narrow therapeutic dose ranges, necessitating the monitoring of serum levels and other functions, such as thyroid and kidney. In either acute or treatment-resistant chronically ill patients, polypharmacy can lead to drug-drug interactions, thereby increasing the potential risk for serious side effects.

Psychiatric Diagnoses

Pay especially close attention to nonpsychiatric medical problems that present with psychiatric symptoms and vice versa. Most DSM-5 (American Psychiatric Association 2013) diagnostic criteria sets include a medical exclusion, requiring that general medical causes be ruled out before a primary psychiatric diagnosis is made. Although perhaps less "exciting," a negative

TABLE 9–1. Screening tests for all hospital patients

Complete blood count

Chemistry panel (i.e., comprehensive metabolic panel)

  Glucose (fasting is ideal)

  Electrolytes

  Renal function tests

  Total creatine kinase

  Liver enzymes

  Albumin

Thyroid-stimulating hormone with or without free thyroxine

Serum pregnancy test (in women of childbearing age)

Urine toxicology screen

Serum level(s) of medication(s) patient is taking (when clinical correlation with level is supported by evidence or there is concern for toxicity)

  Lithium

  Valproate

  Tricyclic antidepressant

or normal test result can be an important piece of evidence that offers reassurance to a patient in distress and opens the door for consideration of a psychiatric disorder.

Laboratory Tests

The concept of "medical clearance" of all potential psychiatric inpatients is controversial, and little evidence supports the extensive screening laboratory studies required by many psychiatric hospitals, free-standing or otherwise, before a patient is admitted. Most experts recommend limiting the general screening panel to a few items appropriate to any general medical screening examination (Table 9–1) and adding more extensive testing only in special populations or in specific patients who require additional workup (Table 9–2).

Brain Imaging

With the development of computed tomography (CT) in the 1970s and especially magnetic resonance imaging (MRI) in the 1980s, the field of psychiatry seemed to be on the brink of having sensitive and specific tests for some diagnoses. Neuroimaging techniques continue to be refined and ad-

TABLE 9–2. Additional diagnosis- and population-based laboratory tests

Diagnosis or population	Laboratory test
Elderly	Vitamin B_{12} level
High-risk behavior (e.g., injection drug use, sexual promiscuity)	Treponemal or nontreponemal test for syphilis
	Hepatitis B virus surface antigen, surface antibody, and core antibody
	Hepatitis C virus antibody
	Nucleic acid amplification testing for gonorrhea or trichomonas
Eating disorder	Electrocardiogram
Antipsychotic prescription	Lipid profile
Cognitive impairment or altered mental status	Neuroimaging
Known medical illness or suspicion of specific illness contributing to symptoms	Diagnosis specific

vanced. Every year more people have routine access to modalities that seemed like science fiction a decade or two ago. Scans are extremely useful research tools, and through the ability to "show something" that is different between groups of patients, they inspire further investigation of underlying physiology and pathology and help "prove" that psychiatric illness is a brain disease. However, as with laboratory studies, the evidence for routine brain imaging in psychiatric patients, even those admitted to the hospital, is lacking. Besides select situations discussed in the following subsections in which a given test can help narrow the differential diagnosis, the yield for screening CT, MRI, or other scans is low. But certain clinical situations do call for serious consideration of an imaging test. A useful way to remember these is to separate them into three categories: general medical (including catatonia and delirium), young adults, and older adults.

Suspicion of a General Medical Etiology

Suspicion of a general medical etiology underlying psychiatric symptoms is aroused when a patient has focal neurological findings on physical examination (e.g., stroke), when some symptoms do not fit the typical pattern (e.g., predominant visual hallucinations in psychotic disorder), when onset is acute (e.g., encephalitis), or in some cases when typically effective treatments seem less so (e.g., medications for acute mania). Depending on the modalities available and the ability of the patient to cooperate, a CT or MRI scan in such a case is reasonable, with the latter usually preferred unless the patient is unable to tolerate several minutes lying still in the scanner. Discussion with the radiologist can be extremely helpful, both to refine the clinical question and to get advice on the most appropriate test to order.

Catatonia and delirium are included under general medical here even though both are frequently seen on consultation-liaison services or can develop while a patient is on the inpatient psychiatric unit. Either can be secondary to general medical or neurological illness, or an adverse effect to medication. Given the potential severity and associated mortality rate with these syndromes, an MRI is typically indicated to evaluate for an identifiable cause or to assess effects on the brain from the condition itself. Electroencephalography also can be helpful, especially differentiating delirium from other causes of altered level of consciousness if the diagnosis is questionable and to add evidence to a case for catatonia.

Young Adults

Young adults constitute a large proportion of psychiatric inpatients because of the typical ages when many mood and thought disorders first present. Especially, for example, in an academic hospital affiliated with a large university, the loss of family structure, experimentation with substances, or the stress of new relationships and academic responsibilities can trigger or exacerbate episodes of illness. Nonspecific abnormalities in these patients are common but rarely contribute to the diagnosis or require an adjustment in treatment. Even so, a large list of metabolic diseases can present in adolescence or young adulthood, many of which have psychiatric symptoms and characteristic imaging findings. A basic MRI scan can be obtained in most facilities with relative ease, so you should have a low threshold to consider a brain MRI for young adult patients who are manifesting any serious mental illness for the first time, particularly one who shows atypical symptoms or has specific medical or neurological findings.

Older Adults

Older adults admitted to the inpatient psychiatric service often present a diagnostic challenge. They may have been living with symptoms for years and have finally lost the ability to cope as a result of a decline in physical health or a change in psychosocial support. They also might be presenting with something new. Late-life depression can have more significant cognitive symptoms and is often associated with vascular risk factors. Given the higher likelihood of neurovascular disease or other brain pathology in this population, consider a brain scan when someone presents with new-onset mood disorder in older age. In terms of dementia, including distinguishing it from delirium or depression and differentiating between types, both standard MRIs and more specialized neuroimaging techniques can be very helpful.

Neuropsychological Tests, Clinician-Rated Scales, and Patient Self-Report Scales

As with laboratory studies and neuroimaging, appropriate deployment of psychometric tests, symptom surveys, and rating scales can bring important information to light that guides diagnosis and treatment. Likewise, indiscriminate testing without formulating thoughtful questions to be answered can be expensive, unhelpful, and stressful for both you and your patient. A dizzying array of tests and scales is available for all kinds of clinical situations. It is important to be familiar with a few basic tests that can be integrated into your daily routine or the unit's admission and patient care workflows to have objective data about a patient's condition and response to treatment. You must also know which consultants are available to your team if more comprehensive evaluation is necessary.

Diagnosis

Diagnosis, although based primarily on history and clinical interview, can be aided by symptom scales or structured questionnaires. Several comprehensive structured interviews have been developed, such as the Structured Clinical Interview for DSM-5 or the Mini-International Neuropsychiatric Interview. Often used in research settings, these can be too long for regular clinical use. But for a complex situation or for a trainee developing diagnostic and interview techniques, they can provide helpful structure. You may find instruments to rate severity of specific syndromes or diagnoses useful in initial and follow-up assessments. For example, in depression, clinician-rated scales like the Montgomery-Åsberg Depression Rating Scale and the Hamilton Depression Rating Scale or patient-rated scales such as the Patient Health Questionnaire and the Beck Depression Inventory can confirm the diagnosis and stratify severity. Scales are also available to help you assess anxiety, substance use, attention-deficit/hyperactivity, impulse control, psychosis, autistic characteristics, disordered eating, trauma, sleep problems, and numerous other clinical situations.

Tests of Cognitive Status

Tests of cognitive status warrant separate discussion given the frequency with which you will encounter patients with obviously altered cognition; decline in ability to function; or concerns about memory, attention, or communication. Many of the illnesses treated in the psychiatric hospital include cognitive deficits, such as "pseudodementia" in severe depression, negative symptoms in schizophrenia, and undiagnosed primary dementia presenting with neuropsychiatric or behavioral symptoms. Furthermore, some of the treatments prescribed, including benzodiazepines and ECT, can have cognitive side effects. Finally, in situations in which a patient's capacity to consent for treatment, or even consent to be in the psychiatric hospital, is a concern, assessment of memory, reasoning, and ability to understand information provided is extremely important.

The Mini-Mental State Examination and the Montreal Cognitive Assessment are two of the most common cognitive screening tests used in hospital settings. Each may be administered by the physician or other staff with appropriate training. They are useful to detect and track broad-based deficits in attention, orientation, and memory. Although limited in both sensitivity and specificity, they are excellent as rapid and easy-to-use tests to detect suspected problems and monitor day-to-day cognitive changes such as might occur with an ECT patient.

Psychological Testing and Neuropsychological Evaluation

Psychological testing and neuropsychological evaluation are more formal options to consider when a deficit is found on screening, the diagnostic picture remains unclear despite other assessments, more comprehensive information is required for subspecialty referral, a pretreatment baseline or posttreatment assessment for ECT is needed, or questions of competency arise. These typically involve consultation with a specialist, with whom you should discuss the reason for testing, clinical question(s), and how the results will be used.

Treatment Response

Treatment response can be tracked with measures that are sensitive enough to detect changes in severity over the relatively short course of most psychiatric admissions. Objective evidence that a patient's condition is improving can be useful as you plan a trajectory toward discharge, reassure a patient or staff members who do not yet see clinical progress, or justify ongoing treatment to administrators or insurance reviewers. This includes suicide rating scales, which are more often used in the office or emergency department to assess the need for admission but also can be used on the inpatient service to track severity of the primary reason a patient needs hospital care.

Medication Management

Pharmacological treatment is an important focus of inpatient psychiatric care. For many hospitalized patients, it is the primary intervention. The proportion of inpatients receiving any psychiatric medication and the proportion of those receiving *multiple* psychiatric medications have grown over the last several decades. Our understanding of what psychiatric medications do and how they do it continues to grow, along with elucidation of the pathology underlying psychiatric illness.

For the typical armamentarium of 15–20 medications, you should have immediate recall of starting and maximum recommended doses, common drug-drug interactions, typical adverse effects, serious adverse effects, appropriate laboratory monitoring (when applicable), and timeline of expected response to medications. More detailed information and characteristics of medications prescribed less often usually can be obtained from an online database.

Two specific areas of focus are especially pertinent for the hospitalist: use of medication to address acute symptoms and initiation of medications that will be continued beyond discharge into follow-up and maintenance care. Details about specific agents are beyond the scope of this section, which focuses on the general approach to and goals of treatment in the context of the inpatient care model. The most common presenting problems for which medication is used on the inpatient psychiatric unit include agitation, psychosis, depression, suicide risk, and mania. The first, agitation, is treated almost exclusively in hospital settings and is addressed in greater detail elsewhere (see Chapter 11, "Acute Disorders").

Psychosis

Psychosis is among the most common reasons for admission to a general inpatient psychiatry unit, depending on the location, the availability of outpatient treatment in the community, and whether the unit accepts involuntary patients. The evolution of antipsychotic medications starting in the 1950s fundamentally changed the work that hospital psychiatrists do. Addition of second-generation antipsychotics to the toolbox through the 1990s and early 2000s resulted in more options with fewer disabling and outwardly visible side effects, but whether efficacy differences exist within or between these groups remains controversial.

Your choice among antipsychotic medications for a psychiatric inpatient usually turns on other variables, including drug-drug interactions, side effects, comorbid medical illness, how quickly a patient might respond to the intervention, and transfer from inpatient treatment to outpatient follow-up. Most of these variables are addressed in all treatment settings, but the last two are more typical of hospital-based care.

Speed of Response

Speed of response to an antipsychotic is not just important when the medication is being used urgently for agitation. Psychosis is often distressing and disabling, and you have a duty to relieve that suffering. For most patients, reintegration into the community as soon as possible is desirable. Inpatient psychiatric beds have become an increasingly precious resource. Payers and hospital administrators monitor length of stay and maintain pressure to provide effective treatment quickly. Your choice of antipsychotic and dosing schedule will affect all of these factors.

The first issues to consider as you choose a medication with time in mind is what the patient is willing to take and what alternatives are available if it is to be administered involuntarily. A medication acceptable to the patient today has an advantage over one that must await a court order. Ease of administration may support a medication that is given once rather than twice daily, that need not be taken with food, or that is available in an orally disintegrating tablet. Consider the rate of dose titration and how much time will be required to reach the target effective dose. These practical issues, far more than minor differences in pharmacokinetics, determine the length of stay.

Continuity of Care

Continuity of care is a critical consideration to improve long-term outcome and avoid readmission. This factor should drive decision-making both at admission and at discharge. At the initiation of treatment, give preference to medication with which the patient is familiar and has previously done well. For the significant proportion of patients who are admitted because they discontinued an effective medication, inquire about the patient's reasons for doing so. If it was side effects or lack of access, consider a change in medication or dose; if it was a less justifiable reason, such as denial of the diagnosis, relapse on substances, or lack of motivation, give preference to the previous medication. Be comfortable negotiating with patients, always staying within the parameters of effective treatment options but not rigidly holding to your preferences.

From the beginning of treatment, consider what things will look like in the first few days after discharge. Continuity of care demands consideration of whether the patient has the financial and personal means to acquire the medication, the follow-up care provider agrees with the treatment plan, and the patient is motivated to continue treatment. These issues will all affect the initial choice of medication.

As you consider what treatment will look like after discharge, project the patient's condition over weeks and months. Will a long-acting injectable medication be preferable to daily dosing? If so, choose an antipsychotic that can be readily transitioned to a depot form. Consider whether that transition allows loading doses or requires an extended period of oral overlap. This long-term perspective from the first day of hospitalization may well make the difference in total days of inpatient care.

Depression and Suicide Risk

Depression, often accompanied by elevated suicide risk, is among the most common reasons for psychiatric admission. Of course, suicidal ideation and suicide attempts are not exclusive to depression, but for the purposes of organizing this section, they are considered together. As with antipsychotics, your choice of antidepressant medication will be influenced by potential drug-drug interactions, side effects, interactions with medical illness, how long it takes to titrate the medication to an effective dose, and likelihood of the patient continuing the medication after discharge.

The conventional wisdom that antidepressants "take 4–6 weeks to work" has been challenged in the last decade or so. Recent studies make the case that some of the improvement experienced by medication responders can be observed in the first several days and much more improvement over the first 1–2 weeks (Mitchell 2006; Taylor et al. 2006). Thus, rather than limiting your observations to whether the patient's initial doses cause side effects, it may be reasonable that a patient could have measurable relief from symptoms of depression even during a brief stay. Moreover, ECT can rapidly relieve symptoms of severe depression (ECT is discussed further in the "Electroconvulsive Therapy" section later in this chapter).

In addition to the broader issue of depression, depending on a patient's diagnosis, situation, and medication history, consider a pharmacological or other somatic intervention specifically aimed at suicide risk. Substantial evidence indicates that lithium is protective against suicide, especially in bipolar disorder but in unipolar depression as well. In patients with schizophrenia, clozapine not only is recognized to be the most effective medication but also has antisuicide properties. ECT, as discussed later in this chapter, can reduce suicidal thoughts and intent over just the first few treatments.

Mania

Mania is a less common but acute and potentially dangerous condition that requires aggressive pharmacological intervention in the psychiatric hospital. As with managing psychosis, your familiarity with short-term effects of medications and availability of different routes of administration are important, and patient preferences, outpatient plans, and a view to longitudinal treatment will all inform your treatment decisions.

The standard of care involves combined treatment with a mood stabilizer (e.g., lithium or divalproex) plus a second-generation antipsychotic. Addition of a benzodiazepine, especially when a less-sedating antipsychotic is used, can be helpful. Divalproex requires no dose titration, achieving therapeutic serum levels in a few days. This is tolerated as well as more gradual dosing and works as well as or better than other options. Lithium, although usually started at a modest dose, can be titrated quickly to achieve therapeutic levels and take advantage of its calming properties.

One major advantage to managing mania on an inpatient service is the opportunity for close observation and frequent assessments of therapeutic response and side effects. Sleep, frequency of aggressive or intrusive behaviors, and pressured speech are readily observed and fairly reliable measures of elevated mood. Even under ideal conditions, manic episodes typically take 1–2 weeks to show significant improvement. Careful monitoring allows you to discern whether progress is occurring even before symptoms have significantly resolved, thereby avoiding unnecessary changes in medications or avoidable polypharmacy.

Individual and Group Therapy

Medications constitute only one component of effective inpatient treatment, albeit the one with which psychiatrists have the most direct responsibility. It is essential, however, that you be skillful in the application of psychotherapies, if not in their conduct then at least in their incorporation into the treatment plan. Many of these are appropriately combined with daily team rounds in which a variety of issues may be discussed. The two primary goals are 1) to bring immediate clinical benefit to your patients and 2) to assess your patient's capacity for and interest in different therapies that may be part of a follow-up course of outpatient treatment. These "auditions" of psychotherapy options greatly facilitate discharge and follow-up planning.

Supportive Therapy

Implicit in every patient interaction is the need to empathize and establish a therapeutic relationship with your patient. Patients benefit from the structured nature of the inpatient unit, benign interactions with staff, the installation of hope implicit in their seeking care, and a sense of being heard and understood. All staff are involved in these interactions and thus contribute to a therapeutic environment and the patient's care. Psychiatrists, generally cast in the role of team leader, are especially valued when they engage patients in these ways.

Even if only a few minutes are available, take time to listen to your patients and interact in a genuine and open way. Allow yourself to share their experience of their environment, stressors, and symptoms. Convey appropriate optimism without overpromising or disregarding real and insoluble problems. Set aside technique for relationship, at least for a moment each day. Frame all interventions in the larger context of their lives rather than the narrow confines of their diagnosis. Medical students are particularly well positioned to do this; with few tools beyond their concern and time, they are often cited as the most important components of a patient's hospital stay.

Problem Solving

Real lives include real problems, some of which may have been directly responsible for a visit to the emergency department or stay in the hospital. A few of those problems can be addressed concretely, including school issues, housing, stressful work environments, or legal entanglements. Social workers may assist in connecting patients with financial entitlements, such as Social Security, veterans' benefits, or other disability payments. School officials are often open to discussion of class requirements, schedule extensions, examination postponements, or other direct interventions with faculty. Housing may be stabilized as finances are regulated. Assistance with legal issues may be arranged. For more global, ongoing stressors such as family conflict, meetings with family to directly discuss and address issues may be helpful.

For some of these issues, such as family meetings, a psychiatrist may be especially helpful, and you may consider direct participation. For others, such as establishment of disability, your involvement will be more administrative, filling out forms or writing letters. In all cases, your awareness and attention during team and patient interactions play a key role in their success.

Patient and Family Education

Few things are as frightening or disorienting to a patient or family member as the onset of a major psychiatric disorder. Responses such as disbelief, minimization, catastrophic thinking, anger, and fear are common, distressing, and rarely helpful in dealing with the symptoms of a newly diagnosed condition. A compassionate but frank discussion of your opinions regarding the diagnosis, etiology, appropriate treatment, and prognosis are critical to address those issues and may make the difference between acceptance and treatment adherence and denial and rejection of treatment. For an initial diagnosis, your involvement in those discussions will add weight and depth to the opinions and recommendations that other team members may have already tried to share. Participate in at least one of those meetings. Listen to the patient's and family's concerns and questions. Gather additional background information from family. Provide as much information and clarity as possible. Be candid about the limits of what you know and what you are certain about. Involve social work staff and trainees and transfer some of your authority to them in the meeting. Let them continue to process, and get involved again if new issues or questions arise.

Cognitive-Behavioral Therapy

Although typically performed over a course of 12–20 individual or group sessions in outpatient clinics, cognitive-behavioral therapy (CBT) lends itself well even to the short stays of most hospital settings, albeit with some modifications. With the configuration of the CBT group changing daily, there is little opportunity for the relationships typical of other groups to develop, making personal sharing and peer support less prominent. The therapist also cannot build a therapeutic relationship over time. With those limitations in mind, patient education about common disorders (usually anxiety and depression) and the use of specific tools and strategies (e.g., cognitive restructuring and relaxation) becomes the primary intervention. Often, lists of tools, such as deep breathing and self-guided imagery, will be distributed and patients encouraged to practice them outside of the groups.

Most of these groups will be conducted by social work, nursing, or activity therapy staff rather than the physician, but your awareness of the content of the sessions will allow you to incorporate and reinforce developing skills in your daily discussions with patients. They will be a useful alternative to "as-needed" medications that may not be available after they leave the hospital.

Dialectical Behavior Therapy

The emphasis in dialectical behavior therapy (DBT) on classroom-style groups, focused modules, and multiple discrete skills used makes it an ideal therapy for hospitalized patients. Although nominally designed for patients with borderline personality disorder, many of its skills are useful generally, and any cognitively intact and motivated patient may benefit. The skills taught in DBT groups are readily applied, may be beneficial even with little practice, and are easy to reinforce during other interactions with physician, nursing, social work, and activity staff.

You may also find DBT a useful adjunct to your own wellness and that of other staff members. Concepts such as mindfulness and interpersonal effectiveness are of such benefit generally that we offer them to staff as well as to patients (in separate venues) with positive results.

Motivational Interviewing

A recent addition to the therapeutic techniques appropriate to the hospital setting is motivational interviewing. In contrast to CBT and DBT, this modality is especially appropriate for the physician and may facilitate progress when a patient's desire and willingness to move forward are absent or have stalled. The fundamental principle of motivational interviewing is to allow patients to identify their own priorities and goals and then to help them explore the obstacles they have faced in meeting them. The focus must be kept on the patient's internal issues rather than outside factors, with gentle guidance toward an understanding of what changes need to occur. Although most popular in the hospital for patients not yet willing to seek substance use treatment, motivational interviewing is equally effective with other issues, such as medication adherence or participation in psychotherapy. Key elements are to approach the session with patience and an open mind, allow the patient time to reflect, and wait for the patient to come to the realization of the need for change and the direction it should take.

Activity Therapy

Engagement in arts and crafts, games, and other entertaining activities seems at first glance to be trivial ways of filling time but serves several important functions in both evaluation and treatment of patients. The ability of these activities to distract a distressed and overwhelmed patient is immediately apparent, but less often appreciated is the implicit message that such distraction is a legitimate therapeutic tool the patient can use both now and later. In addition, skilled activity therapy staff have the opportunity to observe and assess a patient's capacity to maintain attention, organize a project, use strategy, and interact constructively with staff and peers. These observations have high predictive value for patient functioning after discharge. Communicate the importance of these activities to your patients. Review the detailed progress notes prepared by activity therapy staff and include them in daily team meetings.

Psychodynamic Psychotherapy

Most aspects of psychodynamic therapy are reserved for long-term therapeutic relationships, whether in outpatient or in residential treatment settings. Many of the same processes are in play during acute admissions, however, and your attention to them may facilitate both assessment and treatment of a significant number of patients. You need only invite a psychodynamically trained colleague to join you for teaching rounds periodically and observe the effect of a psychoanalytic interview on your patients to appreciate its value. As hospitalists, we tend to focus on efficiency, diagnostic clarity, and actionable pathology in our assessments. We routinely recognize biological risk factors and mechanisms, the role of environmental stressors, and persistent patterns of pathology, but we are often less attuned to unconscious processes and motivations, immediate manifestations of transference and countertransference, or the multiple and complex functions of symptoms. You need not harbor vain aspirations to conduct in-depth psychodynamic therapy during a depressed and suicidal patient's 5-day hospitalization to gain and share insights that will affect the course of treatment as much as initiation of an antidepressant.

Electroconvulsive Therapy

ECT, which has been administered to patients with severe psychiatric illness for more than 80 years, remains the gold standard intervention for the most severe depression, especially when the patient's life is in danger from suicidal ideation, difficulty with self-care, or poor nutrition. ECT is especially effective for both psychotic depression and mood-congruent psychotic symptoms in elderly patients. A second major indication for which ECT is clearly the go-to treatment when medications have failed is catatonia. Although most often secondary to a mood disorder, catatonic symptoms caused by schizophrenia or medical and neurological illness likewise respond well to ECT.

Secondary indications for ECT include treatment-refractory psychosis in patients with schizophrenia (for best results, ECT should be combined with clozapine), mania, self-injurious behavior comorbid with autism spectrum disorders, and neuroleptic malignant syndrome, which shares some characteristics with catatonia. Occasionally, referrals are made to the ECT service for severe and medication-refractory Parkinson's disease, unrelenting tardive dyskinesia, and even status epilepticus when all other measures have failed to terminate the seizure.

Typically, ECT is performed in a hospital setting, where the anesthesia requirements for the procedure can most easily be met in a dedicated ECT suite, the postanesthesia care unit, or an operating room. Inpatients will usually be away from their hospital unit only an hour or two, after which they can safely return to rest or participate in the treatment program. Outpatients constitute a growing segment of patients receiving ECT, coming to appointments from home, where they will return the same day.

A common patient statement heard by ECT providers is, "I wish I had done this treatment sooner!" As a psychiatric hospitalist, whether part of the ECT team or not, you are uniquely positioned to alleviate suffering and save lives by making timely referrals for ECT when indicated. Although we often see patients at one of the worst times in their lives, the overlap between common reasons for admission to the psychiatric hospital and conditions for which ECT is effective offers an opportunity.

The ubiquity of depression and utility of ECT in the hospital setting make it one of the procedures that hospital psychiatrists most often add to their personal training and armamentarium (see Chapter 4, "Training and Background"). ECT-credentialed physicians should be on every hospital staff, accustomed to working with the most severely ill patients. Their role includes preparation of the patient for ECT by optimizing the psychiatric medication regimen (e.g., by removing anticonvulsant medications); recommending further pre-ECT diagnostic workup such as for patients with cardiac or pulmonary disease; and scheduling the ECT treatments so as to minimize disruption to the overall inpatient plan (e.g., administering ECT to inpatients early in the morning).

Some patients, such as fragile elderly individuals or those with concerning medical comorbidities, might be seen initially by an ECT psychiatrist in the outpatient clinic but then will be admitted to the hospital to perform ECT more safely. Furthermore, although it is frowned on to admit someone or keep a patient in the hospital for "psychosocial" reasons or convenience, in certain situations, the patient simply does not have the social support to have ECT as an outpatient, and inpatient ECT is the only way to access needed treatment. The care and support available on the inpatient psychiatric unit are an invaluable part of a successful ECT course in all of these situations. It is especially satisfying when a patient improves enough with inpatient ECT that he or she can be discharged home to finish the course as an outpatient.

Although ECT effectively alleviates depression, suicidal ideation, and other symptoms relatively quickly compared with other treatment options, length-of-stay studies indicate that a course of ECT results in longer hospitalizations, even when data are adjusted for diagnosis and illness severity (Olfson et al. 1998). This can lead to some tension if length of stay is a metric by which you and the service are evaluated, even though research also shows that definitive treatment with ECT, assuming the patient responds and is able to continue with maintenance ECT, decreases readmission rates, yet another example of the need to balance risks and benefits and pros and cons in an individual patient's treatment plan (Ross et al. 2018).

KEY POINTS

- Medical assessment of psychiatric inpatients includes general medical screening and specific testing when appropriate indicators are present.

- Formal instruments that score specific symptoms, such as depression or memory impairment, are useful adjuncts in diagnostic assessment and can track the progress of symptoms during treatment.

- Psychotropic medications used in acute care settings should be chosen not only for their short-term tolerability and speed of response but also for their appropriateness after discharge.

- Psychosocial interventions, including individual and group psychotherapies, problem solving, and activity therapy, should be included in all acute hospitalizations.

- Electroconvulsive therapy is a safe and effective treatment that is highly beneficial for many otherwise unresponsive mood disorders, catatonia, and other conditions.

References

American Psychiatric Association: Diagnostic and Statistical Manual of Mental Disorders, 5th Edition. Arlington, VA, American Psychiatric Association, 2013

Mitchell AJ: Two-week delay in onset of action of antidepressants: new evidence. Br J Psychiatry 188:105–106, 2006 16449694

Olfson M, Marcus S, Sackheim HA, et al: Use of ECT for the inpatient treatment of recurrent major depression. Am J Psychiatry 55:22–29, 1998 9433334

Ross EL, Zivin K, Maixner DF: Cost-effectiveness of electroconvulsive therapy vs pharmacotherapy/psychotherapy for treatment-resistant depression in the United States. JAMA Psychiatry 75:713–722, 2018 29800956

Taylor MJ, Freemantle N, Geddes JR, Bhagwagar Z: Early onset of selective serotonin reuptake inhibitor antidepressant action: systematic review and meta-analysis. Arch Gen Psychiatry 63:1217–1223, 2006 17088502

CHAPTER 10

Guidelines, Algorithms, and Order Sets

Michael D. Jibson, M.D., Ph.D.

Treatment of psychiatric disorders
requires a balance between individualized care and standardized therapy. Without question, the patient's personal experience of illness, preferences for care setting and type, and responses to treatment must be taken into account in any clinical encounter. Within the hospital setting, however, several factors argue in favor of greater attention to evidence-based practices and standardized care than may be prevalent in outpatient venues. Among these are the acuity of symptoms present, the need for rapid and definitive treatment, payer expectations, and the frequency of changes in care provider over the course of a hospital stay or even an emergency department visit. Within this context, clarity about best practices and consistency across providers are essential.

Role of Evidence-Based Medicine

The practice of evidence-based medicine may be defined simply as a willingness to base a clinical decision on randomized controlled studies rather than on personal experience. The primary strengths of evidence-based evaluations and treatments are their reproducibility and defensibility. By definition, high-quality studies provide clear outcomes that will be largely unchanged each time a study is done with a similar population under comparable conditions. Most medication efficacy studies include a substantial portion of hospitalized patients, making their findings especially applicable in this setting. Furthermore, during the hospitalization, other aspects of a patient's condition are closely monitored and controlled, just as they are in most drug trials. Nowhere would it be more likely to find patients responding exactly as they do in these studies. In part for these reasons, evidence-based practices are most useful in cases of inpatients beginning new therapy, outpatient providers anticipating follow-up care, and payers committed to good outcomes efficiently achieved.

Limits of Evidence-Based Medicine

Even the best evidence, however, tends to be narrowly focused and of limited applicability to individual cases. Well-conducted clinical trials are intentionally designed to obscure individual differences in favor of probabilities applicable to large populations. Despite optimistic predictions and hyperbolic claims to the contrary, there is scant basis to predict what treatment will be most effective for any single patient. Treatment choice remains a process of informed, but uncertain, risk. Efficacy trials have the additional disadvantage of being based on uncomplicated cases, with deliberate exclusion of even the most common comorbidities or complicating factors. Real-world "effectiveness" studies, in which a treatment is tried in patients and conditions more typical of actual clinical settings, are less common and do little to address personal differences in response.

Moreover, high-quality evidence of any kind is a rare commodity, leaving the field to wring the tailings of limited studies into meta-analytic vats in the hope that some new truth will emerge or to turn to groups of experts for whatever wisdom they may converge on. The optimistically defined concept of *best practices* is composed of these useful but limited resources.

Meta-analyses allow statistical assessment of larger groups of patients than single studies, which may help blunt the effects of specific issues within individual trials, but they are limited to existing data sets and are often populated by a preponderance of studies intended by their sponsors to find a specific outcome. They require arbitrary decisions about which studies will be included and usually require trials involving different durations, doses, and even outcome measures to be combined into a single analysis. Finally, the number and certainty of the conclusions drawn from meta-analyses are highly dependent on the credence of the authors.

Expert guidelines are likewise produced by a wide range of processes, ranging from things as ephemeral as the insights of a single practitioner with more experience than peers to a theoretician postulating novel or secondary mechanisms of action for a drug or psychotherapy. Somewhat more credible are guidelines prepared by a small group of self-selected and like-minded individuals discoursing on their perspectives. Most defensible are systematic and formal consensus processes involving peer-selected experts basing their recommendations on a combination of familiarity with pertinent research and extensive clinical experience. Not surprisingly, the less formally derived guidelines tend to offer great specificity in their recommendations, whereas the more formal recommendations are vaguer and more general. All of the guidelines are limited in the validity of their recommendations. Some include an assessment of the quality of each recommendation, on the basis of how good the underlying evidence might be and how strong the consensus among the experts is. In doing so, they primarily demonstrate that a decided minority of the final recommendations boast high-quality evidence to support them.

Advantages of Evidence-Based Medicine

Perhaps the strongest justification for the use of these flawed tools is that the alternative is a single physician basing decisions on personal clinical experience, overlooking the problems of limited sample size, nonrandomized treatment selection, open-label assessment of responses, and confirmation bias in the interpretation of results. The effects of two to three consecutive cases of successful or unsuccessful treatment with a new medication or other therapy preclude the considerable act of faith required to trust a formal study or follow a guideline that predicts a different outcome in most patients. In practice, most physicians succumb in some degree to the excessive salience of their personal cases. Of even greater concern is the individual clinician whose career follows a course of diagnostic and therapeutic drift, developing idiosyncratic patterns of seeing a narrow range of pathologies in a broad range of cases and using unique and characteristic therapies driven more by the psychiatrist's predilections than the patient's problems.

The appropriate role of clinical experience lies in the skilled establishment and use of a therapeutic relationship, appreciation for diagnostic limitations and nuance, and recognition of when a prescribed course of therapy is on track or needs to be changed. Clinical experience that can be trusted to guide treatments and outcomes requires tens of years and thousands of cases. It should be recognized by peers before it is assumed for oneself. It includes acknowledgment of one's limitations and a hunger for new and better data, not a disregard for it. True clinical wisdom is the judicious combination of both of these elements in patient care.

The role of evidence-based medicine, in contrast, is to form the foundation on which clinical experience and skill are built. It guides the novice practitioner through early clinical decisions. It defines the default evaluation and treatment options for routine cases and the starting point for the decision to deviate from those norms. It requires specific justification for a different choice, preferably based on additional evidence or at least a tangible rationale. Appropriate bases for moving away from an accepted guideline for a specific patient include a previous failed trial, concern about specific symptoms or side effects, cost and availability of a test or treatment, pertinent comorbidities, or patient preference. Inappropriate reasons include recent advertising, anecdotal recommendations, informal (and unregulated) drug trials, unsubstantiated models of the drug's mechanism of action, and in most cases the physician's personal experience.

On hospital services, evidence-based decisions have additional benefits. The severity and urgency of many cases drive the need for definitive assessment and rapid, effective treatment. Peer-reviewed evidence is the best guide to select the highest-yield treatment for such cases. It allows treatment to begin more promptly by empowering on-call or weekend staff to move forward rather than waiting for the "regular team" to convene. It gives confidence to nursing staff that a proven and familiar treatment is in place. It minimizes the likelihood of a transition in the treatment plan when a new team arrives on the service over subsequent days.

Payers are the designated villains in too many hospital vignettes and have absorbed endless criticism in debates about the high cost of medical care. In truth, insurers have the greatest stake in containing health care costs and have demonstrated admirable restraint and foresight in their demands on providers. As champions of evidence-based care, they are more often derided for encouraging physicians to follow the data than for denying payment for their doing so. Physicians who follow accepted evidence and reputable guidelines are far more strongly positioned to defend the treatment they provide than are those who argue in favor of the supremacy of their own expertise. In this instance, at least, the providers and the payers should be on the same page. Strength of evidence is one of the primary factors used by payers in determining the critical issues of patient copayments and duration of hospital-based care authorized for reimbursement. This policy is not an arbitrary restriction, but a legitimate expectation to ensure the most efficient use of health care funds.

One unfortunate consequence of the recent focus on physician fatigue as a cause of medical errors is an increasing number of transitions in care during hospital stays. Shorter physician hours lead directly to more physicians involved in each case. In contrast to the situation in which multiple specialists convene to discuss a case, however, the sequential involvement of numerous physicians carries significant risk not only for communication errors but also for diffusion of responsibility for treatment planning or frequent changes in treatment based on each practitioner's personal preference. Use of evidence-based algorithms or guidelines offers one option to address these latter issues. With all hospital-based medical staff basing decisions on the same body of data, a consistent and predictable course of therapy can be implemented at the outset of the hospital stay, and each subsequent decision can be made in the context of that plan.

Vignette

Dr. M was an experienced and capable inpatient psychiatrist accustomed to treatment of high-acuity patients. She was a frequent invited speaker at continuing medical education programs and worked hard to stay abreast of research studies and formal guidelines as they became available, promptly incorporating them into her treatment. As a holiday weekend approached, a severely manic patient was admitted following his failure to adhere to treatment over the past few months. After an appropriate initial evaluation, including a review of records, contact with outside providers, and interviews with the patient and his family, Dr. M restarted the patient's previous regimen of olanzapine and valproic acid at moderate doses with a plan to titrate the drugs over the course of the next few days back to the patient's previous levels. She ordered lorazepam as an adjunct for agitation and insomnia.

Over the 3-day weekend, three different attending psychiatrists completed rounds on the service during the day, and two different residents covered the service overnight. Dr. N noted disapprovingly on Saturday that the patient had shown little improvement after 36 hours on the regimen and was not comfortable with olanzapine, because it had caused too many metabolic problems in his own patients to justify its continued use. He switched the patient to aripiprazole, starting at a low dose to avoid akathisia that he had witnessed in another patient. That night, the nursing staff paged the on-call resident because the patient still was not sleeping after 2 mg of lorazepam, receiving an order for trazodone as the primary sedative thereafter. On Sunday, the patient was acutely agitated, leading Dr. O to add chlorpromazine, a drug that had been her favorite during residency two decades previously because it invariably "brings these patients down." The patient still did not sleep that night and received a trazodone dose increase. On Monday, Dr. P noted that the patient had a distant history of alcohol use disorder and discontinued lorazepam. He was appalled by the use of an antiquated drug like chlorpromazine and an ineffective agent like aripiprazole, neither of which he had ever found effective in his own patients, and started risperidone, with injectable ziprasidone as a backup if the patient required as-needed medication, which he did that night.

Dr. M returned on Tuesday to find her patient in restraints, the family enraged, and the staff desperate for more effective treatment. Dr. M reimplemented the original treatment plan, increased the availability of lorazepam, and educated staff about the expected course of treatment response in a manic episode. As she had predicted, within a few days, the patient had calmed down and was well on his way to recovery.

Even with all its limitations, the incorporation of evidence-based guidelines and treatments is essential to optimize hospital care. It does not preclude the need for clinical experience but rather supports and informs it. Properly incorporated, it is the best alternative to provide consistent, high-quality treatment.

Practice Guidelines and Algorithms

Beyond the commitment of individual clinicians to stay abreast of pertinent research and recommendations, specific measures can be put in place to promote this process. Practice guidelines from a variety of sources are available to cover a broad range of clinical situations. A few of these include more specific algorithms to guide the clinician through sequential steps of treatment.

Externally Generated Guidelines

Numerous professional organizations have produced treatment guidelines and recommendations of varying quality and reliability. The American Psychiatric Association has been particularly active in publishing treatment guidelines, several of which are available on the organization's public website (www.psychiatry.org/psychiatrists/practice/clinical-practice-guidelines), with additional guidelines under development. These guidelines are among the most conservative in their pursuit of both evidence and consensus of experts, with rigorous standards for who participates in the process, what studies are included, and how specific guidelines are reached. As a consequence, the guidelines probably represent the best such materials that can be created at the time of their publication. The downside of this exhaustive process is that specific recommendations tend to be vague and general, often with explicit acknowledgments that adequate data to justify more directive steps are not available. They each leave ample room for individualized treatment, but not always with recommendations to guide the clinician beyond first steps. Less experienced practitioners find the absence of specificity in the guidelines a limiting factor. Perhaps their most useful function is to define the minimum standards of care for the targeted disorders.

Government agencies have contributed to the development of several more practical and specific guidelines, including the National Institute of Mental Health (NIMH)– and U.S. Agency for Healthcare Research and Quality–sponsored Patient Outcomes Research Team recommendations; the expert consensus Texas Medication Algorithm Project for schizophrenia, bipolar disorder, and depression; the empirically derived NIMH Sequenced Treatment Alternatives to Relieve Depression study; and the thoroughly manualized National Institute for Health and Care Excellence UK guidelines. Each of these has the advantages of input from recognized experts in the field, a focus on practical issues and interventions, and incorporation of the highest quality data available. Each suffers from the same difficulties faced by the professional organizations, and most quickly go out of date with the introduction of new medications at a more rapid pace than the authors could accommodate.

Commercially available print texts, such as *The Maudsley Prescribing Guidelines in Psychiatry* (Taylor et al. 2018), and electronic references, such as DynaMed (www.dynamed.com), Epocrates (www.epocrates.com), Medscape (www.medscape.com), and Up-to-Date (www.wolterskluwer.com/en/solutions/uptodate), provide more practical and specific recommendations generated by internally selected and paid experts and peer reviewers. These publishers tolerate a higher level of uncertainty regarding the evidence that informs their guidelines in order to provide at least some concrete direction to clinicians who may be encountering a disorder with which they are less familiar. The great advantage of these resources is the rate with which they can be updated, with frequent print editions and the electronic resources undergoing revision every few months.

Each of these guidelines has its place in directing clinicians toward a more rational and systematic approach to patient care. None has resolved the issues of uncertainty and randomness in treatment selection. Consequently, none has become the standard of care for any psychiatric disorder.

In addition to directing a practicing psychiatrist toward the most defensible treatment options, guidelines and algorithms play a critical role in education. In contrast to the uncertainty experienced by a trainee trying to synthesize a treatment decision from a large body of divergent information or, worse, receiving conflicting recommendations from different faculty supervisors, a clear and specific guideline is an ideal way to begin to make these decisions. With standardized default choices, the basis for individual differences can be highlighted. Any decision to deviate from the guidelines requires a specific rationale that will serve as the basis for discussion with the supervisor, providing additional learning opportunities.

From an education perspective, the disadvantage of these tools is that they make it possible for an unmotivated trainee to implement treatment without doing any thinking at all. Herein lies the role for the supervisor, who should be constantly probing for understanding with questions about the basis for every decision, including those on the guidelines, with their advantages and disadvantages. The question "Why that decision?" should be asked frequently and always as a neutral query, not an accusation. Any answer that begins "In my clinical experience..." must be confronted and redirected to a pertinent body of evidence.

Internally Generated Guidelines

Local institutions have occasionally filled this lack of a universal standard of treatment with guidelines produced exclusively for their own use. These have varying degrees of evidence to support them but have the practical advantages of being specific, available, and appropriate for local needs. They are an exercise in standardization over optimization, giving greater weight to consistency across providers and settings than to nuances in efficacy or tolerability among treatments. They most often reflect the preferences of a few senior practitioners but are often informed by the same data, if not the same rigorous methodology, as the more formal guidelines.

Vignette

After having to intervene in several disputes among hospital services over who should provide initial treatment for intoxicated patients with other medical or psychiatric problems, Dr. Q, the chief of clinical service for the hospital, convened a work group to establish a protocol for alcohol detoxification that could be done safely on any unit by physicians and nurses with a wide range of training and experience. The work group included representatives from all of the major services, but none had a dominant voice, and they quickly realized that their work would never get done without compromise. The group agreed that despite evidence that longer-acting benzodiazepines had advantages in some patients, they would use only lorazepam because its straightforward metabolism, low dependence on liver function, and multiple routes of administration would be appropriate in a wider range of settings. The timing of doses was based strictly on pharmacokinetics and required a separate physician order to increase the frequency of administration. The trigger for dosing was limited to specific physical examination and vital sign parameters rather than subjective patient reports. Use of adjunctive antipsychotic medications required psychiatric consultation. None of the services was entirely happy with the resulting "treatment by committee" or the intended consequence that all would share in the care of these patients. The medical teams bristled that their authority as experts had been undermined, the surgeons were incensed that obviously psychotic patients would be treated on their services without high doses of intravenous halo-peridol, and the psychiatrists were not pleased by the prospect of avoidable consultations.

When implemented, however, the advantages of standardization soon proved decisive. The protocol was available as a single "order set" that could be implemented with a few keystrokes, making it instantly popular with house officers. Nurses quickly learned the routines involved and appreciated the clarity of parameters. The number of adverse events related to withdrawal steadily declined, as did the number of withdrawal-related consultations, and lengths of stay were reduced by having patients on the appropriate services even as they went through detoxification. The protocol was soon embraced throughout the medical center, despite its limited adherence to individual bits of evidence.

Regulatory Requirements and Guidelines

A specific subcategory of guidelines consists of those generated not by professional organizations or expert consensus but by regulatory agencies, payers, or medical center administration. Typically intended to address specific problems or enhance overall quality of care, these regulations tend to be specific in their expectations but general in their application, affecting a large cross-section of the hospital in an attempt to avoid rare but catastrophic errors (e.g., "sentinel events" in Joint Commission parlance), to ensure that contracted care is actually provided, or to nudge statistical measures in a more favorable direction by bringing about small changes in numerous occurrences (e.g., better average scores on patient satisfaction surveys).

Credentialing and Oversight Regulations

The number and complexity of rules and guidelines governing hospital services are sufficient to necessitate the existence of entire offices devoted solely to compliance with their expectations. Indeed, *compliance* is now a stand-alone concept requiring no further clarification, encompassing issues of honesty, transparency, and responsibility in financial matters but also in other areas of regulatory oversight. Within medicine, it includes issues of billing legitimacy, accuracy and security of medical records, and maintenance of patient confidentiality. Violation of compliance standards by individuals may result in civil and occasionally criminal penalties not only against the individual perpetrator but also against the medical center. Consequently, both individual clinicians and hospital administrators have a responsibility to ensure that compliance standards are consistently met. At the level of the physician, these requirements are handled through three primary mechanisms: education, standardized procedures, and oversight.

Education

Education typically takes the form of orientation materials and refresher courses at regular intervals. This approach is primarily useful for those whose native inclination is to follow the rules and whose integrity is internally driven but who benefit from direction regarding how best to direct those qualities of character. This is particularly true in areas of patient confidentiality and the integrity of the medical record, in which clinicians unburdened by guile may act in good faith to serve their patients by disclosing information to family members or by using their access to medical records to share reassuring information with close friends without formal consent from the patient. Education is highly effective in clarifying the limitations on such activities and preventing incidental violations.

Standardized Procedures

Standardized procedures are likewise most useful for well-disposed individuals who need occasional reminders of the prescribed order of things. Examples include nursing staff being required to see a medication consent form in the chart before administering a drug, unit clerks checking patient authorization forms before allowing visitors on an inpatient service, and electronic medical records providing warnings about audit trails before allowing access to a chart. These procedures are helpful but at the cost of time and attention through their pervasive repetition.

Among the most common of these warnings are "pop-ups" and "alerts" built into the electronic medical record. These automated warnings often block further actions in the chart or order system until they are addressed. Examples include a reminder to check lipid levels whenever an antipsychotic medication is ordered, a request for an explanation whenever duplicate or overlapping medications are ordered, or a reminder that a patient restraint order will soon expire. The positive aspect of these notifications is that they ensure attention to specific details that must not be overlooked. The negative side is that they soon become repetitive and tiresome in settings where they are frequent and the clinical staff are familiar with the issues involved. "Alert fatigue" is the name given to situations in which alarms become so common that they are routinely ignored or circumvented rather than addressed. It may have the paradoxical effect of making clinicians less, rather than more, attentive to their content.

Optimal use of standardized procedures involves careful selection of issues to address and use of efficient mechanisms that disrupt the flow of work as little as possible. The more sophisticated electronic record and order systems are ideal for this type of arrangement, although it may be necessary to spend some time with system managers to optimize procedures.

Oversight

Oversight is the final security measure to ensure compliance with these regulations. Audit trails in medical records serve as a powerful disincentive to surreptitious access to charts, as well as providing protection against false accusations of unauthorized pursuit of information. Random reviews of consent forms, as well as rigorous investigation of complaints, provide assurance to regulatory bodies that prescribed procedures are followed. Most of these measures are implemented at the institutional level, and the practitioner need only be familiar and compliant with them.

Vignette

Dr. R was annoyed to be stopped every time he made an adjustment to the antipsychotic medication dose of his agitated and unstable schizophrenia patient. With every dose or frequency adjustment, including one-time orders, a warning popped up to remind him to check the glucose and lipid levels of the patient. Although it took only a few seconds to select a response from a pull-down menu, the process was distracting and frustrating in a setting that was already stressful and demanding. On several occasions with previous patients, he had taken an extra minute or so to jump from the order function to the laboratory results to confirm that this had already been done, each time finding that it was part of the admission routine, further increasing his disdain for the process. One of his residents confided that the line "MD is aware" on the pull-down menu was an effective work-around, which Dr. R was soon using freely. This worked well until a patient taking olanzapine complained of chest pain requiring medical intervention, and the consulting service pointed out that no lipid measurements had been made during the admission. Dr. R contacted the department's medical record representative, Dr. S, who reviewed the problem and set the alert to trigger only if more than a month had passed since the last laboratory test. With this simple intervention, the alerts became far less frequent and provided Dr. R with a useful reminder when they occurred.

Payer Expectations

Most clinical care settings have some measure of accountability to financial overseers who either underwrite or reimburse for patient care. Although not directly intended to do so, their standards constitute an important set of guidelines for how care is provided and documented. In most hospitals, clinical notes are reviewed every few days to establish issues such as patient acuity, clinical need, and level of service before payment for care is authorized. In any setting where such an arrangement exists, clinicians do well to be cognizant of these expectations and the basis on which their funding is provided.

Patient Acuity

Patient acuity is a measure of the intensity of care required to ensure the safety of a patient and clinical staff and the level of intervention that will be required for treatment to be effective. Although most frequently used as a measure of how much nursing or other staff time is required for a patient, it also enters into many payer calculations for reimbursement. In psychiatric settings, documentation of the patient's degree of dangerousness to self or others is the most common basis for determining patient acuity in hospital settings, along with other measures of patient need such as functional disability or emotional distress. Standardized assessments are commonly used by nursing staff to address each of these issues in a systematic way. They also should be reflected in physician notes as a justification for time spent and service provided each day.

Clinical Need

Clinical need refers to the justification for hospitalization, as opposed to outpatient care, for the patient. Although cogent arguments can be made for inpatient care as "optimal" in some cases, both medical costs and ethical preference for care in the least restrictive environment demand that the expense and constraint of hospitalization be avoided whenever possible. Thus, each day of hospitalization must be justified. The most common bases for a hospital stay are to ensure the patient's safety or to provide a supportive environment for patients who are unable to function in a less intensive setting. Most progress note templates include a specific sentence addressing this issue.

Level of Service

Perhaps most dependent on physician documentation is the level of service that will be assigned to each day of contact with the hospital psychiatrist. This is generally based on a complex formula that includes arcane determinants such as how many questions about symptoms are asked, how many mental status items are documented, and whether specific items are assessed. An alternative measure is how many minutes the psychiatrist spends in the care of the patient and what percentage of that time is "care and coordination," as opposed to review of notes and documentation. The ease with which a single documentary oversight can significantly reduce otherwise appropriate reimbursement for care leads many hospital services to include these key items in note templates and to provide frequent feedback from staff in the billing office.

Vignette

Dr. T was a recent residency graduate and addition to the university hospital faculty. She had excelled in residency and was enthusiastically welcomed by the inpatient service. She was a thorough and conscientious clinician who was not hesitant to spend generous time in direct supervision of students and residents, with an emphasis on bedside teaching. Nearly everyone was delighted by her work, but her monthly billing reports showed her amounts well below those of more senior faculty who were actually spending less time on the inpatient unit. One of the "payer liaison" staff from the billing office quickly noted the problem and began sending her daily feedback on why her notes were coded for lower levels of service than other faculty. Most often, the problem was not her care but her failure to document single items, such as "gait and station" in a physical examination and "language" (not just "speech") on the mental status examination, or to change the wording on a stable suicide assessment to clarify that it was actually reviewed and updated each day. With this feedback and adjustments to the template she was using, her reimbursement quickly rose to reflect the quality of work that she had been doing.

Quality Improvement and Patient Safety Measures

Quality improvement and patient safety are discussed in detail in Chapters 15 ("Quality Assessment and Improvement") and 16 ("Patient Safety"). This discussion is limited to the role of guidelines, algorithms, and order sets in facilitating these goals.

In general, the great obstacle to both of these processes is not the identification of areas for attention or the conceptual design of processes that achieve the desired ends but rather implementation of measures that will effectively change clinician and staff behavior. Structured processes are ideal mechanisms for bringing about such changes rapidly and decisively, but sometimes at the cost of efficiency and employee satisfaction.

The practice of medicine includes two fundamentally different arenas of activity. The first consists of the probability-based processes of diagnosis and treatment planning. These are conducted in a world defined by *P* values and confidence limits, with no reasonable expectation of certainty. This is especially true in psychiatry, which is distinguished (somewhat) from the rest of medicine by the absence of "gold standards" for diagnoses beyond the much-debated criterion lists prepared by committee vote for the latest DSM edition. Even a flawless application of these standards can never transcend the inherent uncertainty of the method by which the standards were set. In a world of 95% confidence intervals, perfect performance means a perfect 5% error rate. This goal is best achieved via the educational and algorithmic methods already described earlier in this chapter.

The second set of activities, in contrast, may reasonably aspire to 100% effectiveness. These are the processes of implementation of assessment and treatment. It will never be possible to achieve 100% predictive value for a suicide safety assessment, a diagnosis of PTSD, or the efficacy of risperidone in a patient with psychotic symptoms, but it is possible to reach 100% compliance with the completion of a risk assessment, adherence to accepted diagnostic criteria, and delivery of the prescribed medication and dose to the correct patient. These latter processes are greatly facilitated by the transition of guidelines to regulations and of order sets to electronic "hard stops" and required procedures. These tools should be used routinely for appropriate activities, with realistic expectations of their outcomes. The role of the psychiatric hospitalist in this process is to define which processes fall into which category and what outcomes may reasonably be targeted.

Vignette

Dr. V was the director of psychiatric emergency services for a large urban medical center. Widely respected as a conscientious and skilled clinician, he was asked to consult with a work group convened by the medical center director to address the occurrence of 150 completed suicides among patients throughout the hospital system, which was given a charge to reduce that number by 50% within 3 years. Noting that the medical system was responsible for 1.5 million active patients, Dr. V calculated that the expected number of suicides within this population was more than 200 and recognized that even ideally conducted mental health care had limits in this area. Rather than set a goal that was based on factors over which the health system had limited control, he recommended that they define the components of high-quality, evidence-based care and take steps to ensure that they were implemented. Among these were safety screening instruments to more effectively identify medical patients who might benefit from a psychiatric assessment, adequately staffed psychiatric emergency services to provide prompt evaluation, mandatory documentation of a safety risk assessment in all psychiatric emergency department notes, required telephone follow-up of all visits within 72 hours and missed initial appointments, and a standard of 7 days between the emergency department visit and the first outpatient appointment. Each of these was enforced via the electronic medical record, with overrides requiring clear justification. Although none of these met the standard of "evidence-based" or were proven effective interventions, they were reasonable quality improvement measures that represented best practices and could be measured accurately to assess their effect.

KEY POINTS

- Evidence-based medicine is the preferential use of published data rather than personal experience in clinical decision-making.

- Evidence-based medicine has especially important benefits in hospital-based care, where consistency among providers, efficiency in identification of definitive treatment, and clarity of treatment planning are essential.

- Algorithms and guidelines are useful mechanisms to encourage evidence-based care and are readily incorporated into electronic medical records available in most hospital systems.

- Internally generated guidelines and order sets are efficient and useful tools in hospital settings, where patient flow and acuity are high and specific patient issues occur with frequency, such as treatment of alcohol withdrawal, acute agitation, delirium, and suicidal ideation.

- Education, standardized procedures, and regular oversight are critical tools to ensure that services provided meet regulatory standards and payer expectations.

- Structured processes are ideal mechanisms for bringing about quality improvement and patient safety measures in medical systems.

Reference

Taylor DM, Barnes TRE, Young AH: The Maudsley Prescribing Guidelines in Psychiatry, 13th Edition. Hoboken, NJ, Wiley, 2018

CHAPTER 11
Acute Disorders

Heidi Combs, M.D., M.S.
Paul R. Borghesani, M.D., Ph.D.

Acute events occur frequently in inpatient settings and fall under the purview of the psychiatric hospitalist. Among the most important include agitation and violence, delirium and other confusional states, and medication side effects. Early assessment is key to determine the cause and allow for timely intervention and better patient outcomes. Your ability to address these issues is critical to your success in hospital-based psychiatry.

Agitation and Violence

Agitation

Agitation is one of the most common conditions you will evaluate as a hospitalist. It can range from mild to severe and quickly escalate to violence. *Agitation* is a term used to describe both an internal feeling state and physical behaviors. It can present in many ways and is associated with both medical and psychiatric conditions. For some patients, agitation is expressed by a change in affective state. Patients may present as anxious, tense, frustrated, angry, or irritable. Other patients will express agitation through behavior. They may pace, talk faster or louder than usual, gesture more, appear more animated in interactions, or storm around in their surroundings. Finally, agitation can be expressed as heightened reactivity to stimuli, both internal and external. Early identification, evaluation, and intervention are crucial.

Etiology

Many conditions, including medical, psychiatric, and environmental, can lead to agitation (Table 11–1). For most patients, agitation will be the result of a combination of factors. An understanding of the cause of the agitation informs appropriate intervention.

Evaluation

It is important to investigate potential contributing factors as soon as a patient begins showing signs of agitation. Depending on the level of agitation, you may be able to speak with the patient directly. Sometimes all of the information you need can be provided by the patient. Other times patients' level of agitation may preclude them as an initial source of information. Staff often will be able to provide key information, including when the agitation first began, if there were any identifiable triggers, what the milieu was like, if this has occurred previously, how intense the agitation was, and how long it lasted. It is helpful to gather this information from staff when agitated patients do not have insight into their behavior. Other information to review includes laboratory values, vital signs, medications, history of current illness including diagnoses and reason for admission, and history of agitation or violence. A review of the medication list should include medications prescribed, any recent changes, refused medication doses, and as-needed medication use. The goal of your evaluation is to generate a hypothesis for the cause of the agitation.

Nonpharmacological Interventions

To the degree possible, etiology of the agitation determines the intervention. If it is due to a medical cause, such as delirium, a full medical evaluation and treatment of the cause of delirium are indicated. De-escalation techniques would be of little use in this situation. Low-level agitation may resolve without any intervention other than unobtrusive monitoring. A loop back to the patient once the agitation passes may help to identify why the episode happened and what could be done to avoid future episodes. For most patients, however, the appropriate next step is engaging in de-escalation.

De-escalation is a method to reduce distress, agitation, and violence. The basic components include listening to the patient, finding a way to respond that agrees with or validates the patient's position, and offering choices the

TABLE 11–1. Etiologies of agitation

Environmental	Psychiatric diagnosis
High stimulus	Catatonia
Lack of privacy	Mood disorders
Conflicts with other patients	Personality disorders
Instrumental	Psychotic disorders
Intentional behavior to get needs met	PTSD
Medication related	**Substance related**
Side effects	Intoxication
Toxicity	Withdrawal
Medical conditions	
Catatonia	
CNS infection	
Delirium	
Hyperthyroidism/thyroid storm	
Hypo- or hyperglycemia	
Hypo- or hypernatremia	
Seizure	
Stroke	
Traumatic brain injury	

patient can do. Before initiating a conversation with the patient, it is key to estimate the likelihood that the interaction may escalate. If the level of agitation and likelihood of escalation is low, then it may be best for you to approach the patient alone with staff aware and nearby. If the likelihood is anything other than low, then both staff and public safety officers should be present. In these situations, you provide the members of the team a synopsis of the current situation and the plans for next steps. If the level of agitation is high or the patient is demonstrating violence, public safety officers may take the lead. The American Association for Emergency Psychiatry recommends several specific steps for de-escalation (Richmond et al. 2012).

1. *Physical considerations*—When approaching the patient, be cognizant of the environment. Alert other team members that you are approaching the patient. Respect the patient's personal space, and reduce external stimulation when possible. Position yourself with access to the door for easy egress without blocking the patient's access, and if appropriate, leave the door open to reduce the feeling of being trapped.

2. *Verbal skills*—Address the patient by name, and introduce yourself by name in a reassuring, calm tone. If the patient is yelling, lower your volume. Use words like *we* to establish collaboration, and avoid terms like *you need to*, *no*, and *why*. Use neutral words that separate the problem from the individual; ask open-ended questions; use repetition, short sentences, and simple words; and address one concept at a time.

3. *Nonverbal skills*—Use an open body posture, including positioning your body at an angle to the patient's rather than directly opposite, using nonsustained direct eye contact, tipping head slightly to one side, and placing arms just in front of the body with palms open and rotated toward the patient.

4. *Identification of patients' wants and needs*—Simple issues the patient brings up may be easy to address. More importantly, even small choices give the patient more sense of control over the situation. Try to understand whether the patient's agitation was the result of a specific issue or is a general change in mood and cognition.

5. *Active listening*—Express understanding of the patient's issues and perspective. Gently clarify ambiguous comments. Review and summarize the patient's statements.

6. *Agreeing with the patient as much as possible*—Acknowledge legitimate aspects of the patient's concerns.

7. *Setting limits*—Identify the behavior that is unacceptable and why, and help the patient to find an alternative, and reinforce that as a better choice.

Pharmacological Interventions

If de-escalation is unsuccessful, the next step may be administration of benzodiazepines or antipsychotics. For agitation due to alcohol withdrawal, agitated catatonia, or stimulant toxicity, benzodiazepines are the treatment of choice. If the agitation is driven by psychosis or mood elevation, then antipsychotics will be effective both to calm the symptoms and to address the underlying etiology. Second-generation antipsychotics are preferred over first-generation medications because of similar efficacy with reduced motor side effects. Medication administration should occur early if other measures have been unsuccessful in reducing agitation to reduce risk of escalation to violence.

Violence

It is estimated that up to a third of psychiatric inpatients have violent behavior during hospitalization. Violence can be directed at themselves, other patients, or staff. The single best predictor of future violence is past violent behavior, but many risk factors must be considered (Table 11–2). Violence

TABLE 11–2. Factors contributing to violence

Historical/static	**Staff-related**
Previous violence	Younger age
Multiple psychiatric admissions	Less experience
Younger age	Less training about violence
Frontal lobe deficits	Staff setting limits
Dementia	**Environment-related**
Substance use	Overcrowded unit
History of childhood physical abuse	Physically restrictive unit
History of parental substance abuse disorder	Excessive sensory stimulation
	Boredom
History of parental psychiatric illness	Lack of privacy
History of violent suicide attempt	Shift change, particularly swing shift
Current state	
Involuntary status	Medication times
Substance intoxication	Mealtimes
Substance withdrawal	
Psychomotor agitation	
Anger	
Irritability	
Verbal or physical threats	
Akathisia	
Impulsivity	
Pain	
Delirium	
Sleep issues	
Command auditory hallucinations	
Paranoia	

Source.   Adapted with modification from Fischer 2016.

in the inpatient setting can be divided into three categories: impulsivity-driven, psychosis-driven, and predatory.

Impulsivity-Driven Violence

Impulsivity-driven violence is the most common etiology for violence, and staff are the most common targets of the aggression. It is associated with emotional hypersensitivity, exaggerated threat perception, hyperreactivity, and autonomic arousal. It can erupt as a reaction to the perceived loss of control and failure of executive function with no consideration of consequences. High-risk times for this type of violence are when staff members attempt to change a patient's behavior or refuse a patient's request. Impulsivity-driven violence is seen with a wide variety of diagnoses, including substance use disorders, schizophrenia, cognitive disorders, ADHD, intermittent explosive disorder, traumatic brain injury, bipolar disorder, depressive disorders, PTSD, and antisocial and borderline personality disorders.

Psychosis-Driven Violence

Psychosis-driven violence is also most often directed at staff and accounts for the smallest number of inpatient assaults. Risk factors include persecutory delusions and command auditory hallucinations. Disorders associated with this type of violence include bipolar disorder, schizophrenia, traumatic brain injury, and dementia.

Predatory Violence

Predatory violence is the most difficult to predict because it often occurs without agitation or anger but rather in the setting of interpersonal conflict or intentional coercion. It is common on inpatient units, and other patients are most often targeted. Antisocial personality and substance use disorders are most often associated with this type of aggression.

The effect of violence cannot be minimized. Staff may experience decreased productivity, reduced job satisfaction, emotional distress, and physical injury when violence occurs. Negative countertransference can easily develop in team members and negatively affect the care of an assaultive patient. As a physician, it is important for you to help all team members keep in mind that the patient is ill and that most of these acts occur when the patient is in a decompensated state. Patients who are the target of violence can experience a disruption in their treatment as well as physical injury. Family members can become angry with team members for not keeping loved ones safe or preventing them from harming others. They can express distrust or disillusionment of the medical profession.

Physical Management

Physical management, including manual restraint, room seclusion, or mechanical restraints, is restricted to cases of threatened or actual violent behavior. In keeping with regulatory and ethical standards of least restrictive treatment possible, physical interventions are used only after verbal deescalation and medication administration have been ineffective. These steps require trained staff and may involve hospital security or public safety officers' assistance (see Chapter 14, "Legal and Ethical Issues," for a detailed discussion of standards for the use of seclusion and restraints).

Delirium and Other Confusional States

You will often be asked to evaluate dramatic changes in mental status in a hospitalized or emergency department patient. Delirium is far more common in hospitalized patients than generally appreciated or acknowledged. Descriptions of altered mental status by nonpsychiatric providers are highly variable, ranging from a near-exhaustive list of a patient's odd and disorganized behaviors to vague statements such as, "They were OK yesterday and now they're not doing so well." An initial chart review may identify a complicated medication list and extensive medical comorbidities. Medical causes of altered mental status are numerous and span nearly all the medical disciplines. Once the myriad of acute typical etiologies (e.g., stroke, intoxication, cardiovascular disease) are ruled out in collaboration with medical colleagues, you are likely left questioning whether this patient is delirious, catatonic, or psychotic. Typically, these conditions are discussed separately and described as clearly distinct. However, it is our clinical opinion, in conjunction with the growing appreciation of catatonia in the clinical setting, that these conditions are often confused by nonpsychiatric providers, leading to misdiagnosis and prolonged hospitalization. In this section, we present an initial approach to assessing patients with altered mental status, focusing on these three major etiologies: delirium, catatonia, and psychosis.

Delirium

Delirium is common in the inpatient setting, and nearly a third of older medical patients will become delirious sometime during their hospital stay. DSM-5 (American Psychiatric Association 2013) defines delirium as an acute change in attention and awareness with an additional disturbance in cognition that is not better explained by a chronic or evolving neurocognitive disorder or severely reduced arousal, as in coma. These criteria suggest that in a patient who is too somnolent, delirium would not be diagnosed. To avoid this potential error, it is recommended that reduced arousal, precluding the assessment of attention, not preclude the diagnosis of delirium. The DSM-5 definition also emphasizes that delirium is the result of a known or suspected physiological condition and should be attributed to some etiology, even if unequivocally establishing the etiology is impossible. The diagnosis of delirium is the starting point of the evaluation and not the end of the consultation.

Delirium has been historically classified into hypoactive, hyperactive, and mixed subtypes. The hypoactive subtype is characterized by unawareness, staring, lethargy, psychomotor retardation, bradyphasia, or aphasia and is thought to account for about 25% of all delirium. The hyperactive subtype presents in the opposite fashion with restlessness, wandering, distractibility, irritability, pressured and loud speech, and general psychomotor agitation. It is thought to be somewhat more common, perhaps accounting for 30% of all delirium. Most commonly, symptoms of both hypoactive and hyperactive delirium are present, necessitating the mixed category.

Etiology and Pathophysiology

Delirium has many etiologies, and the simple "DELIRIUM" mnemonic is recommended (Table 11–3). Clinical suspicion of any individual etiology of delirium should guide further testing. Medications, especially anticholinergic medications, benzodiazepines, corticosteroids, and polypharmacy, are the most frequent causes of delirium, making a careful medication evaluation essential.

Anyone with medical illness requiring hospitalization or surgical intervention is at risk for developing delirium. Other risk factors include impaired vision and hearing, underlying cognitive impairment, acute or chronic pain, polypharmacy, and substance use and withdrawal. Given the complex etiology of delirium, it is unclear if there is a final, common pathophysiology or if underlying varying neural mechanisms are involved. Functional neuroimaging studies suggest that there may be reduced cerebral perfusion, metabolism, and connectivity during delirium. The association of delirium with anticholinergic medications strongly suggests the involvement of cholinergic functioning in delirium, and monoamine excess may contribute in many cases. Inflammatory modulators, either directly or indirectly via inflammation, also may contribute to acute brain dysfunction.

Evaluation and Diagnosis

All patients with delirium and other acute confusional states (e.g., altered mental status) should have a thorough medical evaluation. Laboratory evaluation and other studies should be guided by clinical suspicion, and extensive testing of patients is ill-advised because it can lead to both real complications and false-positive findings. The patient's medical and social history should be established with particular focus on current medications because polypharmacy is the most common etiology for delirium. Estab-

TABLE 11–3. A simplified mnemonic for the underlying pathophysiology of delirium

D	Drugs and toxins, detoxification, deficiencies (thiamine, niacin, B_{12}), and dehydration
E	Endocrinopathies and the environment
L	Liver failure and lack of sleep
I	Infections and infarction (cardiac or cerebral)
R	Renal failure, respiratory (hypoxia, anemia)
I	Intoxication and injury (e.g., traumatic brain injury, tumor)
U	Urinary tract infection
M	Metabolic changes (electrolytes, glucose)

lishing that the altered mental status is acute, and not chronic, is fundamental. History is the single best way to identify chronic psychiatric illnesses, including dementia. Patients with chronic neurocognitive disorders and intellectual disability, unaffected by altered mental status, can be disoriented and unaware of current circumstances with limited or no insight into recent events. They should not manifest with profound impairment in attention and consciousness (although clearly those with moderate to severe cognitive impairment from any etiology can have significant issues with attention).

Common laboratory tests such as a complete blood count; serum electrolyte, serum urea nitrogen, creatinine, and glucose levels; thyroid studies; and urinalysis are nearly always recommended. Creatine kinase levels can indicate muscular damage and are essential in rigid catatonia or if NMS is suspected. Urine toxicology should be obtained if substance use is suspected, and cerebral imaging is warranted if the patient has any focal neurological symptoms or suggestion of neurovascular or traumatic injury. Other commonly ordered studies include a chest radiograph for evaluation of infection or infarction and serum ammonia and liver studies to evaluate hepatic function. In altered mental status, an electroencephalogram (EEG) should be considered for intermittent symptoms or paroxysmal behaviors and is essential for establishing suspected epilepsy. An EEG can be useful for demonstrating a postictal state and nonconvulsive status epilepticus (although it is often normal). Diffuse slowing is associated with delirium, whereas the EEG does not show specific changes in catatonia.

Treatment

Initial treatment focuses on maintenance of general physiological function with fluid administration, oxygen supplementation, and antibiotics with appropriate clinical monitoring. Collaboration with medical and neurological colleagues is essential as prolonged agitation or bradykinesia from any etiology can lead to a myriad of severe physiological abnormalities. Those physically restrained because of agitation can develop rhabdomyolysis and acute cardiorespiratory failure leading to death. Restraints are also associated with the development of deep vein thrombosis and fatal thromboembolism. Fortunately, restraint of less than 24 hours without anticoagulation treatment is not associated with thrombotic illness.

General steps for the treatment of delirium are supportive care, including fluids, nutrition, and behavioral activation, and symptom management with a combination of behavioral strategies (reorientation, frequent staff contact, use of sitters, avoiding restraints, providing eyeglasses and hearing aids, collaboration with family) and pharmacological strategies. Although the U.S. FDA has not approved any medication for the treatment of delirium, several professional organizations, including the American Psychiatric Association and the UK National Institute for Health and Care Excellence, recommend pharmacological management when 1) the patient is in significant distress from symptoms of delirium, 2) the patient poses a safety risk to himself or herself or others, and 3) symptoms of delirium are impeding urgently needed medical treatment.

Although their use remains somewhat controversial, the most widely accepted medication class is second-generation antipsychotics. The clinician can decide which antipsychotic to use because superiority evidence for any one medication is lacking. Advantages of haloperidol include the variety of dosage forms available (oral, intramuscular, and intravenous), its minimal sedating qualities, and lack of anticholinergic properties. Olanzapine is also available in multiple forms (oral, sublingual, intramuscular) but is sedating and has anticholinergic properties. In the acute setting, metabolic effects typically are not of concern; however, some reports suggest that olanzapine may contribute to acute hyperglycemia and development of ketoacidosis, so care should be taken in those with comorbid diabetes. Aripiprazole is an alternative with little sedation and few extrapyramidal symptoms (EPS), but the evidence for its efficacy is less consistent. Quetiapine is often used in those with parkinsonism given its low risk of EPS, but sedation and orthostatic hypotension are concerns, especially in elderly people.

Catatonia

DSM-5 established catatonia as an entity similar to delirium in that it can occur 1) in the context of another mental disorder, 2) as a consequence of a medical illness, or 3) as an unspecified stand-alone diagnosis in which the symptoms of catatonia are present, but the mental or medical etiology is unclear (unspecified catatonia). Catatonia presents as a hyperactive "excited" type, a hypoactive type, or a mix of both. Excited catatonia is characterized by agitation with altered mental status and may lead to severe complications such as hyperthermia and autonomic dysregulation (i.e., malignant catatonia). Hypoactive catatonia is characterized by mutism; staring; immobility; rigidity; and refusal to eat, drink, or interact and is often associated with bizarre symptoms such as echolalia, echopraxia, posturing, mannerisms, and negativism. The incidence of diagnostic symptoms in catatonia varies, with a much greater number of patients having immobility, mutism, staring, and withdrawal (>90%) and far fewer having catalepsy, waxy flexibility, and echophenomena (<30%), with negativism, posturing, and rigidity falling in between. Presence of three or more symptoms is considered diagnostic of catatonia, and any patient demonstrating mutism or immobility should be evaluated for the disorder.

Estimates of the incidence of catatonia vary between studies but are suspected to be approximately 10% on psychiatric inpatient units, with the hypoactive variety being somewhat more common. Historically, catatonia has been considered a manifestation of schizophrenia but is now recognized as often being associated with mood disorders and neurocognitive disorders, including up to 20% of those with autism and older adults with dementia. Catatonia is a risk factor for neuroleptic malignant syndrome (NMS), and immobility and poor activities of daily living can lead to dehydration, malnutrition, infections, pressure ulcers, and deep vein thrombosis.

Etiology and Pathophysiology

The pathophysiology of catatonia is unknown. Its association with dopamine D_2 antagonists (e.g., high-potency typical antipsychotics) suggests that hypoactive dopaminergic signaling may be a factor. Likewise, treatment strategies that use GABAergic facilitation and glutamatergic antagonism suggest that the balance between inhibitory and excitatory signaling may be disrupted. Some hypothesize that an imbalance occurs between ventral emotional centers and dorsal cognitive control, which disrupts the regulation of extreme fear responses including freezing (as seen in hypoactive catatonia) and the fight-or-flight response (as seen in hyperactive catatonia).

Evaluation and Diagnosis

Catatonia has a broad differential. Antipsychotics, both daily forms and long-acting injectables, can be causal. EPS present with bradykinesia, rigidity, and immobility and are often associated with staring and grimacing. However, EPS are not specifically associated with mannerisms, negativism, or the other bizarre neuromuscular symptoms (e.g., *gegenhalten*, *mitgeghen*, waxy flexibility) common in catatonia. Psychomotor agitation seen in catatonia can be mistaken for akathisia, but the latter is not usually a cause of altered mental status. NMS (see "Neuroleptic Malignant Syndrome" subsection later in this chapter) must be differentiated from catatonia and includes autonomic instability and hyperthermia. Neurological conditions that should be considered include akinetic mutism, locked-in syndrome, and the vegetative state, all of which will present with profound bradykinesia and mental status changes but can usually be differentiated by clinical history.

Treatment

Treatment of catatonia involves the provision of basic medical needs and the specific treatment of its symptoms. Medical causes may account for 20%–40% of all catatonia, including various conditions that all have the potential to cause diffuse cerebral dysfunction. These include infectious and autoimmune encephalopathies, metabolic disturbances, trauma, neurodegenerative disorders, anoxia and neurovascular disorders, medications (especially antipsychotics), and withdrawal from sedatives and dopamine agonists. The treatment of all these conditions is beyond the scope of this chapter and should be completed in parallel to specific treatment of catatonia. Hypoactive catatonia is associated with bed sores, urinary retention, flexion contractures, aspiration pneumonia, and pulmonary embolism, especially when restraints are used or mobility is limited. Treatment with subcutaneous heparin or enoxaparin should be considered in these cases. Catatonic patients with poor oral intake can easily become dehydrated and malnourished and thus would require intravenous fluids.

Specific treatment of catatonia targets several different neurotransmitter systems and includes electroconvulsive therapy (ECT). Benzodiazepines, which act on GABAergic inhibitory systems in the brain, are foremost in treatment. Most authors suggest an immediate trial of lorazepam 2 mg PO or IM followed by reassessment and repeat administration of lorazepam in 1–2 hours. It is estimated that upward of 70% of patients with catatonia secondary to a mood disorder will respond to this initial lorazepam challenge. Unfortunately, catatonia secondary to schizophrenia is less easily treated with benzodiazepines (<50% response rate). After an initial challenge, continued daily treatment with benzodiazepines is recommended. It is not unusual to require high doses (>10 mg/day of lorazepam) for several weeks. The duration of treatment is highly variable, and benzodiazepines should be slowly tapered to prevent withdrawal, reduce the risk of seizures, and minimize the likelihood of relapse.

Other medications for catatonia have been reported for individual cases, including the GABAergic agent zolpidem, the *N*-methyl-D-aspartate (NMDA) receptor antagonist memantine, the weak NMDA antagonist and dopaminergic augmenter amantadine, and dopaminergic agents bromocriptine and levodopa, but none has undergone formal clinical trials.

ECT is a safe and highly effective treatment for catatonia that has not adequately resolved with benzodiazepines or has progressed to the point of medical danger. Its major limiting factors are lack of availability and patients' impaired capacity to give informed consent. In spite of these impediments, ECT frequently provides rapid, complete resolution of catatonic symptoms and may be lifesaving in severe or malignant cases.

Psychosis

Psychosis is best defined as an abnormal mental state that involves loss of contact with reality. Although hallucinations and delusions are easily defined as psychotic, many fail to recognize that disorganized thought and behavior are equally suggestive of an underlying psychotic process.

Etiology and Pathophysiology

DSM-5 recognizes numerous etiologies for psychosis, including all the schizophrenia spectrum disorders, major depressive disorder, and bipolar I disorder. In addition, transient psychosis is common in substance intoxication and withdrawal, PTSD, and some personality disorders—most notably, Cluster A personality disorders (paranoid, schizoid, and schizotypal) and borderline personality disorder. Finally, psychosis may occur in major cognitive disorders.

Evaluation and Diagnosis

Psychotic symptoms are common in both delirium and catatonia; thus, it is essential, for several reasons, to screen for and rule out these disorders anytime you are evaluating psychosis. First, these disorders should take precedence over the symptomatic treatment of psychosis. Of course, if psychosis is contributing to agitation and thus interfering with the evaluation and treatment of any medical condition, including delirium and catatonia, it will need to be addressed. Second, the long-term management of delirium, and possibly catatonia, may not involve mental health care at all, whereas any established psychotic disorder should be referred for ongoing mental health care. Finally, *primary* (i.e., not caused by general medical illness) psychosis is a diagnosis of exclusion with limited recommendations for further laboratory testing and evaluations, whereas delirium nearly always and catatonia frequently involve further medical evaluation for optimal treatment and prognosis.

The major factor distinguishing other psychotic processes from delirium and catatonia is the absence of overt changes in consciousness or attention. Aside from the defining characteristics of hallucinations, delusions, and disorganized thinking, sensorium is usually clear and there is little waxing and waning of consciousness. Furthermore, with the notable exception of substance-induced psychotic disorder, in which a drug screen may be positive or vital signs may be demonstrative of withdrawal, physical examination, laboratory tests, and even neuroimaging are typically unremarkable. These tests may be done to exclude other diagnostic possibilities but not to establish a positive diagnosis.

Contextual history provides the most important data to identify the underlying psychotic process. The longitudinal story of the patient's symptoms, as told by the patient, family, or others, will clarify critical defining features such as a history of functional deterioration, recent mood symptoms, or extensive substance use. In the absence of this information, the presenting psychotic symptoms may give hints of the underlying pathology with their paranoid, grandiose, or nihilistic qualities, but these are frequently overlapping and should not be taken as definitive.

Treatment

Fortunately, antipsychotic medications are effective in the acute treatment of these symptoms irrespective of cause. Few data support the selection of antipsychotics based on efficacy, but there are large differences in side effects, pharmacokinetics, and routes of administration. Parameters to keep in mind include the lower risk of EPS and acute dystonic reactions with second-generation drugs; ready availability of olanzapine, ziprasidone, haloperidol, and chlorpromazine for intramuscular injection; ease of administration (but not more rapid absorption) of orally disintegrating olanzapine and risperidone; intravenous formulations of first-generation drugs; and safety of simultaneous injection of haloperidol with lorazepam. Longer-term metabolic effects are rarely an issue in this setting, but possible transitions to maintenance treatment should be considered even in the acute setting.

Psychosis in the context of alcohol or other depressant withdrawal requires special consideration. All types of psychotic symptoms may occur in this setting and are not by themselves indicative of another psychotic disorder. Although antipsychotics may occasionally be helpful, these cases are best managed with aggressive benzodiazepine treatment, and psychotic features will typically resolve together with other withdrawal symptoms.

Medication Side Effects

Psychiatric disorders and use of psychotropic medications are frequent on inpatient medical and surgical units. Side effects from these medications occur commonly, and the risk increases with polypharmacy. Many of these side effects are benign, but some can cause acute distress, agitation, and mental status changes or can be life-threatening.

Common Acute Side Effects of Psychotropic Medications

Akathisia

Akathisia is described as a subjective feeling of restlessness that can lead to significant tension and psychomotor agitation often manifested as stereotypic, nonpurposeful, repetitive movements. Akathisia occurs in about 25% of patients taking antipsychotics, placing it among the most common side effects associated with this class of drugs. Risk is highly correlated with degree of dopamine blockade, making affinity for dopamine D_2 receptors and dose-specific factors predicting its development. Treatment may include a change in dose or antipsychotic or addition of medication to counteract symptoms. When clinically feasible, a reasonable first step is to reduce the antipsychotic dose or switch to a lower-risk antipsychotic. If this not possible or not effective, then additional agents may be needed. Propranolol, clonidine, and benzodiazepines have shown efficacy in reducing physical symptoms and the feeling of agitation. Anticholinergics are sometimes used, but with less formal evidence of effectiveness.

Acute Dystonic Reactions

Acute dystonic reactions are sustained abnormal postures or muscle spasms most often occurring in the cranial, pharyngeal, cervical, and axial muscles. The incidence of acute dystonia is 2%–3%, most often (90%) associated with initiation or rapid dose increases of antipsychotics or with reduction in medications used to treat acute EPS. Manifestations include stiff jaw, dysarthria, dysphagia, oculogyric crisis, pharyngeal spasm that can lead to difficulty breathing, cyanosis, and opisthotonos. Life-threatening laryngospasm is a rare dystonic reaction and a medical emergency. Treatment for acute dystonia typically involves intramuscular administration of an anticholinergic or antihistamine medication. After the acute event, anticholinergic drugs such as benztropine 1–2 mg bid should be used for at least 4–7 days and may be appropriate as long-term prophylactic treatment.

Anticholinergic Toxicity

The classic presentation of anticholinergic toxicity is agitation that progresses into a hyperactive delirium with visual and/or auditory hallucinations. For some patients, a hypoactive or mixed delirium will follow. Dry mucous membranes, blurred vision, photophobia, urinary retention, and constipation are common. Treatment is focused on discontinuation of offending agent(s), environmental adjustments, and benzodiazepines. If the syndrome is severe, clinicians may consider the use of physostigmine, but this level of intervention would require treatment on a medical rather than a psychiatric service.

Rare Serious Side Effects of Psychotropic Medications

Neuroleptic Malignant Syndrome

NMS is a rare (0.01%–0.02%) side effect of antipsychotic medications that classically presents with changes in mental status, muscle rigidity, hyperpyrexia, and autonomic dysfunction. Cases attributing NMS to amoxapine, citalopram, desipramine, lithium, droperidol, metoclopramide, and valproate or abrupt discontinuation of levodopa also have been reported. An estimated 70% of NMS patients initially experience agitated delirium with confusion followed by muscle rigidity then hyperthermia and profuse diaphoresis. The mechanism for NMS is thought to be a sudden pronounced reduction in dopamine activity. Treatment includes withdrawal of the offending agent and supportive therapy, including cooling the patient and aggressive hydration. Although dantrolene and bromocriptine have been widely used, their benefits are questionable, and they may complicate later stages of recovery. ECT has been reported as safe and effective if available but may require an emergency court order in a delirious or an unconscious patient.

Serotonin Syndrome

Serotonin syndrome classically presents with the triad of autonomic hyperactivity, mental status changes, and neuromuscular excitation, commonly accompanied by confusion and agitation. It is typically attributed to a sudden increase in CNS serotonin transmission as a result of reduced serotonin breakdown (e.g., with a monoamine oxidase inhibitor or inhibition of cytochrome P450 [CYP] enzymes CYP2D6 or CYP3A4), reduced reuptake (e.g., with a selective serotonin reuptake inhibitor), and increased serotonin release, usually occurring in combination. Treatment revolves around discontinuation of the serotonergic agent, administration of benzodiazepines, and supportive care.

Dermatological Reactions

Stevens-Johnson syndrome (SJS) is a rare (0.04% of patients) but life-threatening dermatological emergency associated with the use of more than 100 drugs. Features include fever, influenza-like symptoms, and macular skin eruptions, commonly on the mucous membranes, that evolve into bullous targetlike lesions. In the psychiatric setting, valproate, lamotrigine, carbamazepine, phenytoin, sulfa drugs, and ibuprofen are most commonly associated with SJS. The incidence of SJS is highest in the first 2 months of treatment. Within psychiatry, the combination of valproate and carbamazepine has most often been reported in conjunction with SJS, usually during a transition from one drug to the other. Treatment involves withdrawal of the offending agent(s) and careful inpatient medical monitoring.

Hematopoietic Issues

Agranulocytosis is a life-threatening (5% mortality) condition defined as a granulocyte count less than $0.5 \times 10^3/\mu L$. Within psychiatry, clozapine is most commonly associated with agranulocytosis (or severe neutropenia), leading the FDA to require blood counts at intervals of 1–4 weeks throughout treatment. Additional medications that have documented risk include carbamazepine and chlorpromazine and, to a lesser extent, fluphenazine, oxcarbazepine, paliperidone, perphenazine, quetiapine, risperidone, thioridazine, and trifluoperazine. Treatment begins with discontinuation of the causative agent. Antibiotics may be required to prevent or treat infections. Hematopoietic growth factors may be administered if needed.

KEY POINTS

- Agitation can quickly lead to violence and must be promptly addressed.

- Behavioral methods should be used before somatic treatments when approaching an agitated or violent patient.

- Always consider delirium and catatonia when evaluating an agitated patient.

- Psychosis commonly causes agitation but may not warrant extensive medical evaluation if the presentation is most consistent with an established psychiatric diagnosis.

- Keep side effects from psychotropic medications on your radar because they are common and range in severity.

References

American Psychiatric Association: Diagnostic and Statistical Manual of Mental Disorders, 5th Edition. Arlington, VA, American Psychiatric Association, 2013

Fischer K: Inpatient violence. Psychiatr Clin North Am 39(4):567–577, 2016

Richmond JS, Berlin JS, Fishkind AB, et al: Verbal de-escalation of the agitated patient: consensus statement of the American Association for Emergency Psychiatry Project BETA De-Escalation Workgroup. West J Emerg Med 13(1):17–25, 2012

CHAPTER 12

Transitions in Care, Documentation, and Interdisciplinary Communication

Michael D. Jibson, M.D., Ph.D.

A major difference between inpatient and outpatient care is the more frequent need for transitions in care providers, level of care, and type of treatment in the hospital setting. Emergency department visits are transient by nature and nearly always require that you have a plan for continuity of care after discharge. Responsibility for your inpatients' welfare must be handed off and handed back daily, coverage by your peers typically occurs every weekend, and your schedule may include rotations on and off service as frequently as every week or two. The level of care changes at admission, may be revised during hospitalization, and changes again at discharge. The type of treatment, including the selection and use of medications, psychotherapies, and other modalities, is more likely to change during an inpatient stay than at other times. All of these scenarios require your careful attention to the evolving plans and excellent documentation and communication with previous and subsequent caregivers.

Emergency Care

At its most fundamental level, emergency psychiatry is the simplest of all disciplines, with only one primary task for every patient—to keep the patient and everyone else safe—and one critical decision—to admit or not to admit. The simplicity ends there, however, as the perplexity of how to intervene effectively in the life of a suicidal or an acutely agitated patient is reflected in the complexity of the patient's unique mental, emotional, and social life.

Assessment

Entry into an emergency department always constitutes a transition in care, albeit one with a wide range of previous services, from none to intensive outpatient treatment or transfer from another inpatient or emergency facility. First, you must quickly assess the patient and the situation. Pay attention to how the patient arrives, such as walking in, being transported by ambulance, or getting dropped off by police. Note whether the patient required any form of restraint during the trip and, if so, why. Get as much information as possible from those who brought or accompanied the patient. Learn the circumstances that precipitated their contact, determine their legal status (e.g., involuntary or under arrest), and inquire about any issues that arose during the journey in. Observe the patient for evidence of agitation or aggression, such as shouting, cursing, physically acting out, or attempting to flee. Decide on the basis of this information whether the patient is a reasonable safety risk in a standard waiting area or examination room before you attempt an interview. Place the patient in the least restrictive environment compatible with maintenance of safety, which may include a restriction on leaving the facility, room seclusion, or physical restraint.

Conduct a brief, directive interview focused on the critical issues of safety and need for admission. Some contextual information is useful at this stage, but a detailed review of an extensive history or lengthy process of catharsis is not initially appropriate. Listen to the patient's story, but have a low threshold for directive questions to address your primary concerns. Ask specific questions about dangerousness, especially suicidal and homicidal thinking. Take time to explore the duration and intensity of the thoughts, recent plans and actions, and protective factors or intervening events that brought the patient to you rather than to a medical unit or coroner. Many centers now routinely use formal suicidality screening tools that document patients' responses to specific questions and offer interviewers issues to discuss in more detail. The popularity of these instruments has grown despite a persistent lack of evidence for their efficacy, and many hospital systems, regulatory bodies, and payers expect them.

Treatment Planning

For suicidal patients, consider what level of care will be required to maintain their safety immediately and restore them safely to the community. For those whose issues are not about safety per se, but rather intolerable distress or inability to function, consider what services will be required, or would be optimal, to give them relief and restore them to health. At this stage, additional history and even a brief therapeutic intervention may be appropriate. Consider whether this would obviate the need for hospitalization or an outpatient referral before undertaking treatment. If so, then it is reasonable and appropriate to go forward. If the situation will still require an immediate transition and continuity of care, then it is best to defer any intervention to the next stage of treatment.

Transitions Within the Emergency Department

Length of stay in emergency settings is typically measured in hours, but most patients' stays extend across multiple shifts, and they often receive care from rotating nurses, social workers, and physicians. Efficient, accurate, high-value communication among caregivers is essential in this setting. A variety of written and face-to-face handoff tools are available but are only as good as the time, training, and attention of the people who use them.

The first critical element of an effective handoff in the emergency department is that it contain crucial information specific to that setting, including the presenting problem, degree of acuity, safety assessment, legal status, medical issues, treatment offered, and status of plans going forward, with a clear statement regarding what has to happen for the patient to be ready for discharge. Although this information might be reflected in existing documentation, it is unlikely to be as clearly and succinctly stated or as current as a brief, focused handoff note. Without each of these elements, continuity and progress toward discharge will be impaired.

Second, the tool should be standardized and its use monitored. A specific format will ensure that all information is covered and that tasks still to be done are highlighted. Monitored compliance with the tool will communicate to staff its importance and reinforce its regular use.

Third, it must be easy to use, not require excess time or effort, and minimally duplicate other documentation requirements. Staff time is at a premium in all clinical venues but nowhere more so than in the emergency department. The most important component contributing to this goal is selection of material to be included. One sentence describing the presenting problem, one stating the salient history and pertinent mental status finding, and one describing the anticipated plan and where its development stands should suffice for most cases. An additional "to-do" list of issues in progress may be helpful. Most details of the case, specifics of precipitating events, lists of medications, and other minutia can be gleaned from the medical record if needed.

Finally, if possible, the tool should be presented in person with a verbal handoff to appropriately emphasize critical issues. The affect with which information is presented often communicates important information about patient acuity, interaction with staff, and cooperation that is fully expressed in most written reports.

Transition From the Emergency Department

All emergency department care is transitional in nature, and preparation for a prompt transfer out of that setting is inherent throughout the patient's visit. Your management of that transition depends primarily on where the patient will receive care next and the circumstances of the transfer of responsibility.

Discharge to an Inpatient Unit

Discharge to an inpatient unit is appropriate for patients whose safety cannot be maintained in a less restrictive setting, whose care could not reasonably be provided in a less intense environment, or whose course of treatment would be substantially shortened or improved by hospitalization. Most patients should be engaged in a discussion of the costs and benefits of an inpatient stay and given the option of voluntary admission. Involuntary treatment should be considered for that subgroup of patients whose level of dangerousness or disability is incompatible with an immediate return to the community (for more on involuntary treatment, see Chapter 14, "Legal and Ethical Issues").

The transition in care to an inpatient unit requires direct contact with the receiving facility and a comprehensive note regarding the basis for the patient's admission, findings in the emergency department, and legal status. A candid account of issues arising during the evaluation is essential to ensure that the receiving unit is able to provide appropriate care. Legal status must be clearly stated, as well as degree of cooperation with treatment.

Discharge to Outpatient Care

Discharge to outpatient care is the option of choice for patients whose safety and level of function are less significantly threatened. For those already involved in psychiatric treatment with either a primary care physician or a mental health specialist, direct contact with outpatient providers is the preferred option, both to keep them informed of the emergency department visit and to establish a follow-up appointment with a reasonable time frame, usually no more than 7 days away. This transition will generally involve two-way communication, with the outpatient clinician providing pertinent collateral information to the emergency staff and the emergency department sharing details of the issues that precipitated the visit and the plan to address those issues.

For patients not currently engaged in care, the least useful intervention to facilitate continuity of care is to tell them to find an outpatient provider or hand them a list of names of individuals who may not be accepting patients, may be a poor therapeutic match, or may not accept the patients' insurance. Whenever possible, a better option is to set up an initial appointment before the patient leaves the emergency department, making clear what the next step in care will be. The best arrangement, however, is for patients to have direct contact with the new care provider, engage in a brief discussion of their issues, and agree that their working together is viable.

Inpatient Care

Admission Decisions

From the perspective of the receiving psychiatrist, it is imperative that you screen all proposed admissions to your inpatient service, whether they originate in the emergency department, consultation-liaison service, or outpatient clinic. Critical issues include the type of diagnoses and problems your unit is able to serve, the level of acuity you are prepared to handle, whether you are equipped to deal with pertinent medical problems, and whether there is a reasonable expectation that the patient will benefit from the care you can provide. Never open a case without an exit strategy. Acute inpatient units are not ideal settings to house patients with intractable placement issues, insoluble problems, or no available options for outpatient or long-term residential care. Although on some occasions, you will agree to accept a patient outside these parameters because of other considerations, such as a lack of viable alternative placements, these should be kept to a minimum.

Work with your primary referral sources to educate them about the structure and operation of your unit. Let them know in advance what questions you will ask and what criteria you will use in making a decision to accept or reject a prospective patient. Educate your own staff about those same criteria, and take steps to ensure that they are applied uniformly by whoever is taking the calls. If you are unable to accept a patient, specify the basis for the denial. These steps will not only help maintain the integrity of your inpatient program but also build trust between you and your referring facilities.

Admission Procedures

Request an advance copy of the documents that will accompany the patient to your unit, including a note about the current visit, recent medical records, laboratory results, and pertinent legal forms. This will ensure that you have access to this material, strengthen your review process, and avoid any delay in completion of documentation from the sending medical staff. Review the records both for content and for completeness, with special attention to pending laboratory reports, incomplete contacts with outpatient providers, and payer information.

As patients arrive, quickly verify their psychiatric, medical, and legal status to confirm that they are appropriate for the unit. Give nursing staff time to complete their own assessment of the staffing and personnel needs that must be addressed. Allow the patient to get settled into a room and oriented to the unit.

Initial Evaluation

Irrespective of the quality and detail of the accompanying documentation, your assessment of the patient should be thorough and independent. The basis for this expectation is that inpatient admissions most often occur at times of change in a patient's course or in response to a failure of other treatment, making this an ideal time to reevaluate the patient's diagnosis and course of therapy. Referring physicians are often seeking this evaluation as a valued second opinion and appreciate the additional insights or validation of their views that will result. In addition, you need this level of assessment to be fully responsible for the patient's care while on your unit and after discharge until the first follow-up visit.

Conduct your intake assessment systematically and thoroughly, with attention to each element and to the relationship you are establishing in the process. Work to build rapport with your patients, whether voluntary or involuntary. Introduce yourself and the evaluation process clearly and respectfully. Listen to patients' perspectives and concerns. Explain the rationale for what you are doing kindly but frankly. Respond to their issues with genuine empathy and concern. Pay attention to hints in their affect as to the most sensitive or critical areas to explore. Hesitation, tears, anger, or defensiveness in response to questions are clues that may lead you to the central issues.

Elicit your patient's story through open-ended questions and active listening, interrupting only when necessary to keep the story on track and moving forward. Identify the key problems that necessitated admission and that you can address. Explore the contributing factors that gave rise to those problems, both to create context and to evaluate the level of stress that the patient has faced.

Diagnoses facilitate communication, summarize complex groups of symptoms, and satisfy regulatory and payer expectations, but the compelling reasons for making diagnoses are to direct treatment and predict the course of illness. Form a hypothesis as to the diagnoses that best describe the cluster of symptoms experienced by your patient. Test your hypotheses by asking specific questions from DSM criteria lists and following established standards for the disorders. Make the most specific diagnosis that your data allow, but avoid premature closure and include an appropriate differential list of other possibilities.

Gather historical information about past diagnoses, hospitalizations, medications, psychotherapies, suicide attempts, self-injurious behavior, and current or recent caregivers. Explore substance use carefully and thoroughly, both by direct questioning and by use of screening tools. Cover other medical issues in enough detail to inform psychiatric care, including a complete list of current medications and drug allergies. If not already available from other sources, such as a social work or student note, gather social history regarding early family life and relationships, educational and employment history, adult relationships, legal issues, and abuse or trauma. Focus the family history on mental health issues, including major disorders, substance use issues, and attempted or completed suicides.

Conduct a mental status examination that screens for major symptoms and elicits details on the most pertinent issues. Describe the patient's grooming, hygiene, dress, and demeanor. Characterize behavior, including level of psychomotor activation, appropriateness of posture and gestures, abnormal or typical movements, and level of cooperation. Note the rate, volume, amount, richness of content, and peculiarities of speech. Include a description of the three basic dimensions of mood: degree of elevation or depression, anxiety, and anger. Describe both the range and the content of affect. Characterize the degree of organization of thoughts and classify forms of disorganization into tangential, loose, circumstantial, or other types of association. Probe for evidence of auditory, visual, or other hallucinations. Explore possible delusions, including paranoia, grandiosity, and ideas of reference. Conduct a few screening cognitive tests for orientation, memory, and attention, and then do additional tests as indicated by the history and presentation. Assess insight and judgment primarily on the basis of the history presented, with the addition of formal questions when more information is required.

Do a careful safety assessment, exploring both static and modifiable risk factors. Ask about passive thoughts of death, such as wishes not to be alive, fantasies about becoming ill or injured, and rumination about lethal actions. Determine whether the patient has formulated or is obsessively thinking about a specific plan. If so, consider its lethality, availability, and practicality. Inquiry about intent to act, including any steps, however abortive, that the patient may have taken in the direction of an attempt. Discuss the patient's protective factors, including reasons to be alive, important personal relationships, and goals. Consider supports in the patient's life, including family, friends, coworkers, and mental health professionals.

Vignette

Ms. B objected repeatedly to her family's insistence that she be admitted after a visit to the emergency department to address their concerns that she was depressed and suicidal, which she denied. Dr. A allowed her to state her objections, then asked her in a general way to talk about how her life had been going in the last few months. Given this opportunity, Ms. B soon acknowledged a sequence of disappointments and frustrations that had culminated in her losing her job, an important relationship, and her independence when she had to move back in with her family. Noting that her affect shifted on that last point, Dr. A asked Ms. B to tell him more about her relationship with her parents, eliciting a tearful account of her tightly controlled childhood and hard-won independence, which she now experienced as humiliatingly lost. Even so, she denied being seriously suicidal, with only a "passing thought" of overdose. Dr. A guided her through an exploration of this thought. In response to his specific questions about each step, she soon acknowledged having identified a drug to take, checked to see if the bottle was in the medicine cabinet, and poured the pills into her hand to see how many pills there were. The conversation they had in view of this information led to a more meaningful assessment of her suicide risk and a higher level of acceptance and engagement in treatment on her part.

Admission Notes

Your documentation of this initial assessment is probably the single most important source of information for care transitions in both the short and the long term. This comprehensive collection of well-organized facts and observations should include all critical issues in the patient's course since its onset, as well as a clear summary of your understanding of the case up to that point. It will be referred to by all members of the treatment team, consultants, payers, and subsequent care providers in some cases for years to come. Give it the attention and effort that it deserves.

Begin with a succinct identification of the patient by age, gender, relationship status, and pertinent diagnoses. State the specific problem or problems that led to admission. Do not clutter this initial statement with an exhaustive history, list of discarded past diagnoses, or irrelevant medical issues. Beware of automatically populated lists here and elsewhere in the note that indiscriminately bring in long lists of information that have no real bearing on the current situation.

Use the history of current illness to tell the most complete and coherent version of the patient's story that you are able to construct from all sources available to you. If discrepancies are found among sources, highlight that; otherwise, simply present the narrative as a statement of facts as best they could be determined. After the story, systematically describe the patient's symptoms grouped by diagnostic category. Give a qualitative description of the pertinent symptoms. Include pertinent negative diagnoses and syndromes (e.g., manic episodes, panic attacks) that contribute to the overall diagnostic picture. Conclude with observations about the patient's reaction to admission and willingness to participate in treatment.

The psychiatric history may be presented as either a narrative or a series of categories and bullet points. The critical issue is that the information be accurate, complete, and quickly accessible. Important issues to address include the age at onset of mental health issues, their overall course, and previous diagnoses. The treatment history should include both psychotherapies and medications, with brief details about specific medications, doses, durations, and effects. Significant events to report include suicide attempts, self-injurious behaviors, and hospitalizations. Give a detailed report of substance use either here or in a separate section. Specify the drugs, doses, frequency, duration, and consequences over the patient's course.

The social history may be organized by topic or timeline, in narrative or bulleted format. Seek to create a clear picture of early and current relationships, functional capacity over the life span, and factors such as education, employment, finances, social concerns, and legal issues that may affect the patient's symptoms and recovery. Trauma and abuse should be addressed if they occurred at any point or mentioned as pertinent negatives if they did not. Family history is best presented as bulleted lists focusing on first-degree relatives.

Use the mental status examination to given quantitative (e.g., 0–10) or comparative (e.g., mild, moderate, severe) ratings of the symptoms described qualitatively in the history of current illness rather than repeating what was already said. Include pertinent negative symptoms (e.g., hallucinations, delusions, suicidal ideation) here rather than in the narrative.

Your assessment should include a formulation of the case that postulates how a specific set of factors has converged to cause your patient to develop the current symptoms and problems that led to your inpatient unit. Unless your purpose is to work through a difficult differential diagnosis, do not present a summary of how your patient's symptoms meet the DSM criteria for the final diagnosis, which should already be clear from the historical narrative. Instead, consider the case from a variety of perspectives, such as developmental, behavioral, psychodynamic, relational, genetic, and neurobiological, depending on which serves best to clarify the course and inform treatment. The basis for all elements of the treatment plan should be clear from this discussion. Conclude with a clearly stated differential diagnosis.

Your plan should be evidence-based and economically defensible. Take into account the resources and services available to your patient, along with the patient's and family's reasonable preferences. Make sure the overall intent of your plan is clear, as well as the individual steps that you plan to take. Be transparent about your reasoning and decision-making. Include a realistic target discharge date.

Evening and Weekend Cross-Coverage

The range and depth of information included in an admission or consultation note would be overwhelming for a covering physician overnight or on a weekend to search for the key points required to address a narrowly focused issue. Consequently, there is little alternative to the creation of a synopsis of the notes that highlights critical facts and anticipated decisions. These handoff notes have become increasingly valuable as work-hour restrictions and physician wellness initiatives drive hospitals to schedule briefer shifts and more days off for their staff, creating greater frequency in the need for daily and weekly transitions in care. The most important goals of these short-term transfers of responsibility are to anticipate and effectively manage crises that arise and to minimize disruptions and alterations in the treatment plans created by the primary team. These notes are fundamentally different from those used in emergency settings, which facilitate transfers to new caregivers, in that no long-term transfer of responsibility is expected, and major decisions are deferred back to the primary team. Consequently, they usually require a different template to capture the critical information.

The essential elements of these notes begin with a summary of the patient's diagnoses and presenting problems, emphasizing the primary focus of attention. List the major symptoms being addressed, giving the covering physician a clear idea of the patient's current condition to allow detection of any acute changes. State the basic treatment plan and specific steps that are in progress, especially medication changes. Identify past or anticipated problems and preferred responses. Mention any special considerations that may affect interventions made by the covering team, such as a history of substance abuse or adverse responses to common medications. Effective handoff notes must be reviewed daily and updated regularly.

When you are the covering physician, your goal is to maintain safety and facilitate the existing treatment plan. Take care to refer to the handoff notes before making even minor decisions or adjustments to orders. Do not attempt to modify treatment without a compelling reason to do so. Update the handoff note with any issues that arose or changes you made, explaining to the primary team what you did and why.

Team Transitions

Handoff notes to a new team that is taking over care of an inpatient or a consultation-liaison patient differ in several ways from those required for temporary coverage or emergency department transitions. These notes should include greater detail of the clinical case and a more complete explanation of the rationale for the diagnosis and treatment plan. A good rule of thumb is to describe the case at the level required for you to have an informed discussion with the patient's family about the care you are providing.

As you begin the note, summarize both the major elements of the patient's history and the peculiar details unique to the case. Include those details of the psychiatric history that inform your current decisions, especially previous medication trials, substance use, and level of suicide risk. Note critical events in the current course of treatment, such as adverse medication reactions, failed trials, or medical complications. Describe your diagnostic thinking, including issues that have not yet been resolved, such as the role of personality traits, differentiation between manic and schizophrenia episodes, or the role of substances in the development of symptoms. Outline the treatment plan that is in progress and its intended final form, such as the target dose of medications or expected patient placement.

Most patients benefit more from a sustained period of treatment than from the marginal benefits to be derived from frequent changes between similar medications or psychotherapies. As the leader of the receiving team, you should default in most cases to a continuation of the previous treatment plan, even if it does not reflect your personal preferences or the top recommendation on a consensus guideline. You should not, however, allow yourself to be complacent in your handling of an inherited case. Continue to assess the efficacy of treatment and accuracy of diagnoses just as you would a case you had managed from the beginning.

Consultations

Among the major causes of medical error, few are more frequent or cata-strophic than decisions made outside one's area of expertise. When confronted with an issue, even within the field of psychiatry, with which you are not familiar or up to date, have a low threshold for reaching out to a consultant. Even basic medical problems may justify such collaboration, because your general medical skills decline and standards of care evolve since those few months of your postgraduate year–1 medicine rotations.

As you plan your consultation request, clearly formulate your question or need. Broad and vague requests, such as "Please manage the patient's medical problems," will prove less useful than more specific and targeted requests, such as "Please assess the patient's insulin regimen in view of recent hyperglycemia." Discuss the consulting team's recommendations and plan for follow-up. Be prepared to act on the recommendations you receive.

The infrequency with which we seek consultation within the field of psychiatry is to the detriment of our patients. General psychiatrists typically know little about developmental, autism spectrum, or even attention-deficit disorders in adults. Few nonspecialists are skilled in the use of medication-assisted substance use treatment. For the general psychiatrist, experience and expertise are double-edged swords, yielding exceptional knowledge and skill with the patients most often seen but at the expense of declining comfort with other populations.

For all of these reasons, it is good practice to call on peers not only for informal, "curbside" advice but also for formal consultation. The procedure for doing so should be similar to that used for other such requests, with a note in the medical record justifying the consultation, an order in the chart, and an expectation of an appropriate note in response. Among other advantages, this offers legal protection to both parties and provides a basis for the consultant to bill for the service. These consultations are useful at several levels: 1) to provide you with new perspectives and valuable advice, 2) to expand your knowledge base, and 3) to bolster your confidence in your assessments and treatment plans going forward, even when the consultant simply confirms your opinions.

Vignette

Dr. Z, an experienced and well-regarded psychiatrist, had more than 10 years of experience running a high-acuity adult inpatient unit. He initially took in stride the admission of a 25-year-old patient with an intellectual disability and escalating behavior problems that led his parents, with whom he had always lived, to seek admission. Dr. Z soon discovered, however, that his expertise with patients who have psychosis and personality disorders was ill-suited to the case, and both he and the nursing staff felt frustrated and increasingly endangered as the patient's behavioral outbursts became more frequent and violent. In a corridor conversation with a fellow attending, the name of a colleague who had worked for several years with a similar population came up. Dr. Z chatted with her briefly, then requested a formal consultation, which yielded several practical and effective strategies that could be implemented. With these recommendations and periodic follow-up suggestions, the case soon took a more favorable turn, and the patient was stabilized in preparation for a transition to an appropriate residential program.

Discharge

Every transition from an inpatient unit requires a plan for the termination of hospital care and beginning or resumption of care elsewhere. Attention to the nature and timing of both issues is critical to good outcome.

Discharge Planning

Discharge planning begins with the initial evaluation of the patient, which includes identification of the problems that need to be resolved and the expected time course for treatment. Among the benefits of early attention to discharge are that it encourages prompt and frequent communication with outpatient providers, keeps the team focused and moving forward with treatment, and creates realistic expectations for the patient. Rather than imply to the patient that the stay will continue until his or her symptoms have fully resolved, it makes clear that treatment will involve continued care and further progress after he or she leaves. For more on discharge planning, see Chapter 3, "Consultation-Liaison Psychiatry."

Communication With Outpatient Providers

Communication with outpatient providers should occur at admission in the case of patients already in care, then whenever a change in the treatment plan is contemplated, and as soon as a discharge date is finalized. A verbal or email summary of care will facilitate a smooth transfer to a greater degree than a formal discharge summary that may accompany the patient or arrive days later. Especially important considerations in this transfer of care are ongoing issues that require immediate attention or follow-up, such as laboratory values that need to be checked, doses of medication that need to be given at a specific time, or medications that require further dose titration.

Discharge Notes

Discharge notes should contain enough information to preclude a later reader from having to refer to other documentation from that hospitalization to understand the patient's condition at that point in the course of illness. Some of this may reasonably be copied from the admission note, but with adjustment based on later information or perspectives on the case. It is not necessary to compulsively describe every hospital day or step in a medication titration, but significant events that help clarify the diagnosis or might direct future treatment decisions should be included.

Include your final diagnosis. One goal of DSM-5 (American Psychiatric Association 2013) was to encourage clinicians to make specific rather than general diagnoses (e.g., major depressive disorder rather than mood disorder not otherwise specified). One goal of hospitalization is to observe, gather collateral information, and assess the patient's symptoms and course to clarify this issue. Have the courage to come to a diagnosis and state it clearly in the discharge note.

A final mental status examination and safety assessment, including the basis for the decision that discharge is appropriate, must be included. These will prove invaluable in the case of an adverse event, but their major function is to assist the next care provider in determining the frequency and level of care that will be required. Other information to include in the note are the names and doses of all medications, dates and locations of all scheduled follow-up care, and your contact numbers in case of questions.

KEY POINTS

- Most hospital-based treatment is temporary, and transitions in care among hospital services and from the hospital to outpatient clinic are an integral part of the patient's course.

- Assessment, treatment, and documentation in an emergency department should be focused on the safety and welfare of the patient and others involved.

- Transitions within the emergency department are frequent and focused on safety and immediate ongoing issues, including the course of the assessment and plans for discharge.

- Inpatient admissions need to be screened to ensure that the diagnosis, level of acuity, medical comorbidities, and treatment required are appropriate for your unit.

- An inpatient admission note should be a comprehensive review of the patient's past course and current situation, leading to a clear formulation, differential diagnosis, and treatment plan.

- Evening and weekend coverage notes should be succinct and content-rich, with lists of the problems, diagnoses, treatments, probable issues that you anticipate, and your recommended responses.

- Team transitions include a summary of the major issues and the treatment course to that point, along with the treatment plan you have been following.

- Consultations from other specialties or from psychiatric subspecialties are a valuable tool that you should use regularly.

- Discharge planning includes direct communication with follow-up providers, a summary of significant events during hospitalization, and critical issues for follow-up.

Reference

American Psychiatric Association: Diagnostic and Statistical Manual of Mental Disorders, 5th Edition. Arlington, VA, American Psychiatric Association, 2013

CHAPTER 13

Discharge and Transition to Outpatient Care

Stephen Mateka, D.O.
Sarah Mohiuddin, M.D.

Discharge planning and care transitions are an essential part of your plan for each patient you encounter. For this reason, it is essential that discharge planning begin at the time of admission. Nevertheless, physicians do not work in a vacuum. You work within the construct of your particular health system and in the larger construct of the mental health system in your region. In addition, discharge from an acute hospitalization is affected by outside factors, such as your patient's health care insurance or psychosocial supports. As such, your decision-making around discharge is often affected by several factors.

Treatment of acute exacerbations of psychiatric illness comes with inherent risk, including the safety of the patient and of the people around him or her. Your role as the hospitalist is to take safety into consideration as you determine treatment planning to achieve goals of hospitalization, the overall length of stay, and what aftercare setting best meets your patient's needs for gains to translate to the community while mitigating the risk of re-admission. The inpatient setting and the patients that require it naturally consume a significant amount of time, energy, and effort. In this chapter, we highlight the process of progression toward discharge and transition to out-patient care while offering guidance on the numerous factors expected to be considered and accounted for along the way in a psychiatric hospitalization.

Length of Stay

Length of stay in the psychiatric hospital has shortened significantly over the past century. The psychiatric hospitalization shifted from custodial care in the early 1900s to deinstitutionalization and community-based services be-ginning in the early 1960s, with an accompanying decrease in the number of beds and length of stay. In the 1990s, the emergence of managed health care was accompanied by a continuum of care model featuring integrated and comprehensive care with a wide array of inpatient and outpatient services.

Both positive and negative factors have driven these trends. On the pos-itive side, the advent of effective medications, efficient psychotherapies, and a network of community services have made outpatient care an acces-sible and effective option for most patients. On the negative side, the rapid rise in hospital costs, persistent stigma associated with inpatient care, and advocacy for maximization of personal freedom and treatment in the least restrictive setting possible have made hospitalization a less attractive op-tion. Given this convergence of factors, it is not surprising that most hos-pital stays are now 7 days or fewer.

Be aware of these factors and of specific predictors of length of stay as you begin the process of discharge planning. One of the primary drivers of a longer stay is increased severity of psychopathology, as indicated by fac-tors such as involuntary commitment, multiple psychiatric diagnoses, need for physical restraints, poor insight, low level of baseline functioning, med-ical comorbidities, legal problems, substance use, a pattern of treatment noncompliance, or a diagnosis of schizophrenia. Other factors, in contrast, are associated with decreased lengths of stay, including diagnoses of disrup-tive behavior disorders, ADHD, and history of nonpsychotic violence. Be attentive to these issues as you anticipate the timeline required to identify and actualize goals of the hospitalization and preparation for discharge.

Vignette

Mr. T, a 38-year-old man with major depressive disorder, recurrent, mod-erate, was treated as an outpatient with fluoxetine and as-needed alprazolam. He had two previous psychiatric hospitalizations and a remote suicide attempt. He became more depressed and acutely suicidal after losing his job. He was admitted voluntarily to a private stand-alone psychiatric hospital. At admission, he endorsed passive suicidal ideation and denied active suicidal ideation, plan, or intent. On day 2, responding to the supportive environment of the inpatient unit, he denied all types of suicidal ideation. By day 3, his insurance denied coverage for continued hospitalization. Mr. T did not want to risk incurring further hospital costs but expressed concern and had increased anxiety about managing life after the hospital. The multidisciplinary team was aware on admission of his health insurance limitations and had anticipated an abbreviated hospital course. This awareness allowed for creation of a customized safety plan if he became overwhelmed after discharge. Social work was able to assist with guidance for filing unemployment, provide resources for psychotherapy, and reschedule an appointment with his outpatient psychiatrist so that he could be seen within 1 week of discharge.

Critical Versus Optimal Treatment

With the advent of the continuum of care model, the type of care being delivered in the hospital has required recalibration as psychiatric hospitals begin to take care of patients with higher-acuity illness and safety concerns. In theory, clinicians strive for optimal treatment while ensuring that critical treatment standards, mostly focused on safety, are not compromised. Thus, those standards are met when a patient is discharged and is no longer an imminent danger to self or others. The reality is that critical and optimal treatment lay on a continuum. The lack of standardized treatment practices, increased pressure from insurance companies for discharge, and significant variability in resource availability and patients' access to resources have led the inpatient psychiatrist to focus most treatment planning on acute safety as the primary outcome. By contrast, the concept of optimal treatment involves a commitment to a biopsychosocial, multidisciplinary approach focused on improving their overall quality of life, with safety merely the initial goal. Several factors will affect where along this treatment continuum you are able to operate.

Inpatient treatment is one of the most costly and intensive treatment modalities, and patients' need for this level of care is vigilantly monitored. Some insurers base need for treatment on factors such as safety, whereas others have capitations or day limitations on acute stays irrespective of the patient's condition. No insurer allows unlimited hospital days, and few consider what setting is optimal, leaving the patient, family, or hospital to bear the cost of additional hospitalization. Critical treatment may have to suffice when optimal treatment comes at the cost of compromising a patient's financial well-being. The cost-benefit ratio may have more effect than the risk-benefit ratio in dictating your decision to deliver care. There will be situations in which you may deem a patient as nonacute as related to safety but requiring further treatment to optimize function. You may have to forgo these goals in prioritizing the financial health of your patient.

Patients' previous exposure to behavioral health care services will influence the degree to which psychoeducation for the patient and family serves as a significant intervention during the process of stabilization for discharge. Adjustment of the psychopharmacological regimen and continuity of outpatient psychotherapy are interventions more likely to contribute to stabilization when a patient has well-established care in the community. Coordination of care with outside providers is critical for implementing treatment interventions that will significantly contribute to stabilization at discharge.

The availability of outpatient resources influences the threshold for discharge. For instance, if a step-down treatment option is not feasible, you may be more likely to advocate for continued hospitalization to increase the likelihood that the patient can tolerate a significant drop-off in level of monitoring from the inpatient setting. Although the paradigm of care has shifted to the community, limited funding and availability of outpatient services to meet the demand, particularly for patients with higher severity of illness and/or aggressive behavior, may force you to adapt discharge planning to meet patients' needs. If neither an appropriate level of aftercare nor extended hospitalization is possible, then the highest-yield treatment intervention is comprehensive safety planning.

An interplay of several factors clearly affects where along the continuum of care you can operate. The revised conceptualization of acute hospitalization's purpose redefined what constitutes critical and optimal treatment. This is affected by third-party payers, goal setting for discharge, access to outpatient mental health care, and individualized patient psychosocial factors. The decision to focus on optimal versus critical care often evolves over the course of the hospital stay. As you treat patients' critical needs, it is important to identify opportunities to shift toward optimal care within each unique inpatient care setting. Closing the gap between critical and optimal treatment will influence how best to meet patients' behavioral needs as they transition to outpatient care.

Vignette

Ms. J, a 25-year-old single woman, had unspecified depressive disorder and generalized anxiety disorder. She had no previous suicide attempts or psychiatric hospitalizations and was prescribed sertraline by her primary care physician. She had a course of psychotherapy for self-injurious behavior as a teenager after her parents' divorce. She was most recently admitted to an adult inpatient unit after an impulsive overdose at home with approximately 20 tablets of acetaminophen 500 mg after a verbal altercation with her boyfriend over suspected infidelities. Ms. J reported that about 15 minutes after the ingestion, she began to experience abdominal pain and became regretful of her actions. She told her mother, with whom she lives, who called 911. After medical clearance, she was admitted.

The critical treatment goal was reduction of her suicide risk; thus, treatment was focused on safety planning for discharge back into the community. Optimal treatment involved analysis of the events leading up to the suicide attempt and identified multiple cognitive distortions, including fortune-telling, catastrophizing, and accepted helplessness. Ms. J was able to discuss her fears of being unlovable and alone, which stemmed from her parents' divorce. This offered the opportunity to introduce cognitive-behavioral therapy concepts and dialectical behavior therapy skills to improve her insight and resilience and motivate her to participate in outpatient therapy. A focus on optimizing treatment allowed for social work to arrange follow-up, which included a partial hospitalization program to build on the foundation and momentum established in the hospital. Ms. J was also assisted in finding an outpatient psychiatrist and psychotherapist, who both received hospital records that provided a biopsychosocial formulation to help put her presentation into context and guide outpatient treatment. Before discharge, Ms. J expressed gratitude to the multidisciplinary staff for helping her "make sense" of why she made such an impulsive and dangerous decision.

Factors Affecting Discharge

Numerous factors affect your ability to discharge a psychiatric patient from the hospital. In this section, we elaborate on modifiable factors affecting medical decision-making around discharge.

Because of changes in criteria for hospital admission, the patient population in psychiatric hospitals has higher severity of illness than in previous decades. When planning discharge for a patient with acute suicidal ideation, you should be aware that suicidal thought content on admission and suicidal behavior during hospitalization predict increased risk for completed suicide within the first month of discharge, particularly in the first week. This highlights the importance of a focused treatment plan addressing suicidality during the stay and aftercare treatment on discharge. Specific patient populations who are older than 40 years, have illness onset within the past 12 months, have required more than 1 month of hospitalization to stabilize their symptoms, experience an adverse life event within 3 months of admission, and have a primary diagnosis of mood disorder require further attention. Modifiable risk factors for safety include an unplanned discharge, discharge against medical advice, and tentative or delayed (more than 1 week) follow-up care.

Interventions for depression and schizophrenia specifically mitigate risk after discharge because severity of illness in these specific disorders is associated with increased suicide risk. However, each of these diagnostic categories requires a unique treatment plan. In schizophrenia, pharmacological intervention with antipsychotic medications may improve acute symptoms during a short hospital stay. By contrast, pharmacological efficacy for treatment of depression often extends beyond the time constraints of a typical hospitalization. This speaks to the importance of mobilizing social supports and aftercare before discharge.

Patients with aggressive or assaultive behavior and neurodevelopmental disabilities have a chronic safety risk. These patients often periodically require a higher level of care to maintain safety. In these cases, take into account their living situations as you establish a threshold for discharge. Patients being discharged back to long-term treatment settings with professional staff involvement will have additional assistance in maintaining safety outside the hospital. Patients with lower functioning and a higher loss of function at admission may require more intensive intervention during the hospitalization to be ready for discharge.

The effect of psychopathology, housing stability, insurance coverage, and individual hospital criteria for accepting an admission all ultimately affect discharge planning. This often requires mobilization of resources for the patient to return to the community. You need to advocate for patients early and often through collaboration with social work and care management teams during the course of the hospital stay. Awareness of the factors affecting discharge requires a wide lens, and being able to operate with self-efficacy in varied and flawed systems requires a holistic approach to optimize the care of the hospitalized patient.

Vignette

Mr. G, a 63-year-old man, was admitted to a private, stand-alone hospital in an urban setting. He had a psychiatric history of major depressive disorder and alcohol use disorder and was admitted because of active suicidal ideation with a plan and intent to jump off a bridge after he was thrown out of the house by his wife for drinking. Early in the hospitalization course, he showed guarded affect, aggression, and agitation with posturing, likely precipitated by alcohol withdrawal. During this time, he required intramuscular medication and significant verbal de-escalation on multiple occasions to prevent physical management. He completed a chlordiazepoxide taper for alcohol withdrawal and then was able to participate safely within the milieu. Further assessment of behavioral triggers for emotional escalation led to his being more forthcoming about the stressors in his life.

As part of the plan toward transitioning the patient to outpatient follow-up and coordination, Mr. G was permitted to go off unit to attend Alcoholics Anonymous meetings, which connected him to a local Alcoholics Anonymous meeting when discharged back to the community. Mr. G agreed to outpatient individual therapy. After progress in family sessions, he and his wife agreed to outpatient family therapy. The discharge plan included step-down treatment at a partial hospitalization program with a specific dual-diagnosis program. His wife ultimately agreed to allow Mr. G to return to the home contingent on consistent engagement in treatment and maintenance of sobriety. He then was able to be safely discharged home to his wife with a plan to address personal and familial stressors contributing to his presentation.

Follow-Up Planning and Coordination

Optimal follow-up planning and coordination require coupling of inpatient treatment with outpatient programs and services that can meet the needs of a patient after discharge. You are charged with determining an appropriate aftercare setting to meet the patient's needs, none more important than safety. In the subsequent discussion, we offer guidance in navigating the complexity of discharge planning.

Following the improvement of acute psychiatric illness, the establishment of an aftercare plan is an important modifiable factor for risk on discharge. Initiation of discharge planning at the time of admission alleviates pressure to identify a plan for community care transition in the event of an unplanned discharge or discharge against medical advice. Comprehensive psychiatric follow-up after discharge is a well-established protective factor for maintenance of safety. Because outpatient psychiatric resources vary across health systems and geographic regions, it is incumbent on the hospitalist to be familiar with aftercare options local to the area in order to advocate for the optimal aftercare plan for the patient.

Aftercare planning also requires you to account for alternative levels of care, including long- and short-term treatment facilities. When short-term hospitalization is inadequate for safety stabilization, residential treatment facilities and long-term state hospitals are pertinent considerations. Opportunities for a smooth transition to such settings, however, are typically impeded by limited availability and long wait lists. The unit's case manager or social worker is expected to be the primary facilitator, but you can be a pertinent contributor to the process. Early identification of the patient's need for longer-term treatment, beyond acute hospitalization, positions social work to attempt arrangement of transition of care as soon as possible. In addition, it provides you an opportunity to advocate and coordinate care with prospective longer-term settings. When critical stabilization is attained in the acute setting but long-term treatment remains a realistic and optimal option, it is important to arrange an interim aftercare plan between acute discharge and long-term admission.

Transitional programs facilitate gradual reintegration of the psychiatrically hospitalized patient back into the community. The most common iterations of transitional programs are partial hospitalization and intensive outpatient programs. Partial hospitalization programs serve as the immediate step-down from the hospital when a patient requires the most significant support and monitoring to maintain stabilization immediately after discharge. In partial hospitalization programs, patients commonly attend Monday through Friday for 1–2 weeks, during the typical hours of about 8:00 A.M. to 3:00 P.M. Intensive outpatient programs are a less restrictive treatment environment than partial hospitalization, with decreased total weekly contact with behavioral health professionals. The presence of intensive outpatient programs varies by region. Intensive outpatient programs typically provide care 3 days per week for 2–4 weeks. In both partial hospitalization programs and intensive outpatient programs, patients have daily interactions with a therapist and usually weekly interactions with a psychiatrist, unless an acute situation requires further evaluation. If the acutely hospitalized patient does not have a psychiatrist or therapist in the community at time of discharge, transitional programs assist in connecting patients to these services after discharge from their programs.

Discharge from an acute hospitalization directly back to an established outpatient psychiatrist and/or therapist is appropriate when patients have lower psychiatric acuity. Outpatient follow-up is recommended as soon as possible but no more than 2 weeks after discharge. The least intensive level of care after discharge is with a primary care physician instead of a behavioral health provider. This option should be reserved for patients with the lowest acuity whose admission may have been the product of adjustment disorder or if the treatment plan consists of a psychotherapist and a basic psychotropic medication regimen that the general practitioner is comfortable managing.

Follow-up planning and coordination are paramount to the discharge process. If the primary goal of every hospitalization is discharge, then the secondary goal is to have the gains made in the hospital maintained and generalized to outpatient settings. The aforementioned options include psychiatric treatment options along the community continuum of care model. Choice of aftercare is determined by clinically informed decision-making and availability of outpatient resources. The crux of psychiatric hospital discharge criteria is safety, and the presence of continuous aftercare has been shown to significantly reduce mortality. Awareness of outpatient services, coupled with early and continuous assessment of appropriate linkage to outpatient needs, significantly increases the likelihood that the time, effort, and energy expended in delivering care in the hospital will translate to maintenance of safety in the community.

Vignette

Mr. M, a 54-year-old man with a history of schizophrenia and extensive past hospitalizations that typically were precipitated by medication nonadherence, was picked up by police for acting "bizarrely," taken to a suburban community hospital emergency department, and involuntarily admitted to the hospital's adult inpatient psychiatric unit. On admission, he had paranoia, internal preoccupation, and response to internal stimuli. He improved over the next 10 days with risperidone. He was assessed for decision-making capacity and was able to consent to long-acting risperidone injections. The medication was initiated in the hospital, and Mr. M was discharged to a community mental health partial hospitalization program in his county. The hospitalist team coordinated care to continue titration of his medications while he was admitted to the partial hospitalization program. The hospital social work team coordinated with the outpatient program's social work team to establish community residential housing. In this situation, comprehensive and thorough follow-up planning and coordination allowed the opportunity to translate gains made in the hospital to the community.

Readmission

As in all of the topics discussed in this chapter, the issue of readmission requires consideration and integration of multiple factors to understand how and why this occurs. Clinically, psychiatric illness follows a chronic or relapsing-remitting course in a patient population that often requires significant support for treatment adherence. In addition, continuity of treatment after discharge or barriers to access of the desired aftercare can be significant contributors to readmission. Despite a higher level of acuity and severity of psychiatric illness, inpatient stays are constrained by insurance company authorization, leading to pressure on you to discharge as quickly as possible; this approach presents you with a unique challenge to optimize hospital and aftercare treatment planning. We explore identification of patients at greatest risk for readmission and facilitation of aftercare coordination to decrease the occurrence of rehospitalization.

We have already discussed multiple factors that affect readmission. The shifting focus of care to the community has created shortened lengths of stay, focus on critical instead of optimal care, and an increase in admissions because of lack of adequate outpatient resources. Although inpatient hospitalization is conceptualized as part of a continuum of care model, in reality it is fragmented, and the same factors that lead to greater admissions also lead to increased readmissions. Even when factors that impede care are addressed, patients still have chronic diagnoses and behaviors that affect their safety and need for hospitalization.

Several patient-specific factors increase risk for readmission. Psychiatrically hospitalized patients with mood and psychotic disorders are at increased risk for recidivism. Use of antipsychotics is a risk factor for readmission largely because of the severity of the pathology they treat. Patients with severe conduct problems often experience deeply embedded psychosocial stressors resistant to medication and require long-term intense therapeutic and behavioral intervention. The risk of readmission in this patient population is highest within 6–12 months of discharge. A unique population at risk for rehospitalization are patients currently or at risk for becoming homeless. Patients with histories of substance use, physical abuse, antisocial personality disorder, depression, ADHD, PTSD, schizophrenia, and significant obstacles to access follow-up services in the community increase likelihood of homelessness after discharge, and ultimately readmission. Diagnostic clarification assists in identifying at-risk populations and can guide your treatment interventions to reduce the quantity of hospitalizations.

The highest-yield intervention to prevent readmission targets the initial postdischarge period. The first month after discharge incurs the highest risk for readmission, with the likelihood of readmission decreasing significantly 90 days posthospitalization. The benefits of established aftercare to avoid readmission are multifactorial, including prompt attention to severe psychopathology, improved continuity of treatment initiated in the hospital, and frequent evaluations of acute safety and symptom severity. Of note, patients connected with follow-up care have a decreased length of stay if they are readmitted. Interventions to support the transition from the hospital to community living yield lower rates of readmission compared with less intensive follow-up, particularly for homeless populations.

Your awareness of factors influencing readmission will highlight opportunities for intervention and assist you in identifying high-risk populations. Establishing consistent follow-up care in the first 3 months after discharge is the primary intervention at your disposal to combat recurrent hospitalization.

Vignette

Ms. W, a 42-year-old woman who had bipolar I disorder and long-standing cocaine and heroin use, was admitted to a dual-diagnosis unit in a freestanding private psychiatric hospital in a rural setting. Ms. W had five admissions over an 18-month span, with indications ranging from acute suicidal ideation to opiate withdrawal, worsening mania, and acute psychosis after a 5-day binge of cocaine and heroin use. The team, which cared for her over each of these five admissions, was frustrated with repeated relapse of illicit drug use leading to worsening psychiatric illness and, ultimately, repeated readmissions. During her fifth admission, focus was shifted to critical care and identification of opportunities to improve her quality of life. In an effort to combat feelings of cynicism, helplessness, and burnout in staff, discussions were held around goals for quality of life for the patient, which led to decreased frustration in the staff's interactions with the patient. In addition, increased effort was made on work toward an outpatient treatment plan that addressed substance use to decrease risk for relapse.

Conclusion

We have highlighted the factors you must keep in mind during the discharge process and promotion of a stable transition back into the community. The paradigm shift of behavioral health treatment to the continuum of care model has redefined the type of care the hospitalist delivers and the parameters in which he or she operates. The lack of standardization in inpatient psychiatric settings requires the hospitalist to navigate the variability of practice environments, patient populations, desired outcomes, and options for transition to outpatient care. The hospitalist can be empowered by awareness of the factors that structure discharge planning. Anticipating expected length of stay for patients will frame the expectations for how to implement interventions that progress toward treatment goals. Inpatient hospitalization exists on a continuum in which follow-up care serves to ensure safe stabilization in the community. Optimization of discharge planning serves as a conduit to outpatient treatment to help protect against readmission and, most importantly, decrease mortality risk during the most vulnerable moments in the lives of patients. Care delivered in the hospital and during discharge lays the foundation for patient trajectories toward an improved quality of life. You will encounter many unique challenges to discharge planning and transition to outpatient care. In providing appropriate and comprehensive care to patients, you work to balance unmodifiable factors with factors that are amenable to direct intervention to promote an enriching experience of hospital psychiatry and, ultimately, the best outcome for the hospitalized patient.

KEY POINTS

- The revision of psychiatric hospitalization's role in delivering mental health care has significantly shortened length of stay and consequently shifted how you must identify and actualize goals of the hospitalization and aftercare.

- The emergence of the continuum of care model redefined what constitutes critical and optimal treatment during hospitalization, encouraging you to identify opportunities to deliver optimal care beyond acute stabilization.

- Increasing severity of psychopathology in the inpatient setting requires you to become accustomed to factors influencing discharge in order to customize and optimize treatment planning.

- Choice of aftercare is determined by clinically informed decision-making and availability of outpatient resources, which have been shown to significantly reduce mortality during patients' most vulnerable time.

- When making discharge planning efforts to prevent readmission, target the initial 3-month postdischarge period, when recidivism rates are highest.

PART IV
Special Issues

CHAPTER 14
Legal and Ethical Issues

Ahmad Shobassy, M.D.

Working in a hospital setting

requires you to be aware of certain legal and ethical considerations relevant to this career path. Some of these issues are general principles that any psychiatrist should know, but the extent to which these topics arise and the amount of time they consume are significantly greater in a hospital-based practice. Generally, patients seeking emergency or inpatient psychiatric services are doing so because their symptoms are urgent, acute, and severe, often involving the threat of harm to self or others, behavioral dyscontrol, or altered mental capacity. These conditions require special attention to issues such as risk of harm, ability to accept or refuse treatment, need for physical or medical interventions, and possible restrictions on personal freedom. In this chapter, I highlight the legal and ethical issues that are pertinent to functioning as a psychiatrist in a hospital setting.

Ethical and Legal Foundations

Principles of Medical Ethics

The major ethical principles involved in most mental health care are autonomy, beneficence, and paternalism. *Autonomy* is the right of patients to make choices regarding their own care, including decisions to accept or refuse hospitalization, medications, and other interventions. Autonomy is highly valued in most societies, is a founding principle of law in the United States, and takes precedence over other considerations in most medical decision-making.

Beneficence is a duty of physicians to act for the good of patients individually and society as a whole. Beneficence is the primary motivating principle of all medical practice (not, as is often asserted, nonmalfeasance, as in the adage, "First do no harm") and demands that physicians act whenever possible for the benefit of their patients. In most instances, however, physician beneficence must yield to patient autonomy.

Paternalism is neither a right nor a duty but a principle that may affect this balance of power. *Paternalism* is an assumption of superior knowledge, judgment, and right to act, generally on the part of the physician. This principle may tip the scale of decisions in the direction of physician judgment over patient preference and allow beneficence to take precedence over autonomy.

Most of the ethical and legal issues you will encounter in hospital settings involve the interactions of these three principles. They implicitly inform all of the discussions that follow.

Legal Issues and Assumptions

Many of the questions that arise in the context of medical ethics form the basis for legislative and judicial interventions. It is critical that you be aware of both the principles and the assumptions that underlie those actions. In contrast to medical ethics, laws are an attempt to achieve balance among the many rights of individuals. Among these are freedom from unreasonable interference with personal decisions and actions, protection of personal safety, respect for personal and real property, access to government and private institutions, and noninterference with personal beliefs and values. Each of these may be affected by mental disorders and their treatment, making the interaction between psychiatry and law unavoidable.

Within this framework, certain assumptions prevail, with both positive and negative consequences. Some of these differ in telling ways between general medical treatment and psychiatric care. Specifically, laws regarding medical care assume that patients are able to exercise autonomy until proven otherwise, that most patients want routine medical care, and that legal oversight of patient-physician interactions should be minimized. Mental health law, however, generally assumes that patients may not be able to act autonomously and may even need protection, that patients usually do not want and must specifically request mental health care, and that many aspects of this care (including all that occurs in hospital settings) require intense legal scrutiny.

As a consequence, most legal venues have unique sets of laws that pertain only to mental health care and the patients who receive it. These laws are reflected in a variety of issues, including those discussed in the following sections.

Voluntary and Involuntary Treatment

As the name suggests, *voluntary treatment* implies the patient's agreement to medical care, including treatment setting and interventions. *Involuntary treatment*, on the contrary, implies that some aspects of treatment are taking place without the patient's consent and sometimes against the patient's will. Consistent with the principle of autonomy, voluntary treatment is the rule for medical interventions, whereas involuntary treatment is the exception. Yet examples of involuntary treatment are seen across the various medical health specialties.

In this regard, mental health is no different, and involuntary treatment is pursued only under specific circumstances. Generally, patients with mental health conditions enjoy the right to make choices about their treatment options, including the choice of no treatment. Patients may refuse to participate in mental health treatment for different reasons, including stigma associated with mental illness, poor insight into existing symptoms, and individual socioeconomic barriers. However, because of the safety concerns that occasionally can be associated with mental health, involuntary treatment may be essential to protect the patient and the community from imminent danger.

Voluntary Psychiatric Treatment

Patients who enter the hospital seeking voluntary psychiatric treatment decide for themselves whether to accept the recommended treatment setting, medication, psychotherapy, and other treatments or to exercise the option of no treatment. Even after beginning therapy, these patients have the right to totally or partially disengage from treatment or to withhold consent at any time.

Voluntary hospitalization requires that the patient first be interested in treatment and second be able to consent for it. Voluntary inpatient treatment may best accommodate patients who are seeking help because they have had suicidal thinking, severe symptoms of any kind, inability to function because of their symptoms, or failure of treatment in less intensive settings.

Involuntary Psychiatric Treatment

Involuntary inpatient psychiatric treatment includes restriction of a patient's right to leave the facility and to refuse treatment. Under involuntary treatment, the patient is either opposed to some or all treatment aspects or is unable to consent to voluntary treatment. For the latter and given that some patients desire the treatment but are unable to consent for it, "unconsented treatment" rather than "involuntary treatment" may be more accurate. Involuntary treatment is not limited to the inpatient setting; many states allow for involuntary outpatient care, and the judicial system may mandate some patients to undergo therapy such as substance abuse treatment or anger management counseling during incarceration. Only the issues directly relevant to the role of the psychiatric hospitalist are discussed here.

The involuntary process involves "civil commitment," a judicial procedure to ensure that any limitation of rights meets strictly defined legal criteria. It is launched following the determination that the threshold for involuntary commitment is met and only when the patient declines or is deemed unable to consent for voluntary inpatient treatment. Once the process is initiated, the patient's ability to leave the unit is blocked, access to objects that can be used as weapons will be eliminated, safe transportation to the admitting facility will be arranged, and the required legal documents will be completed. During this initial period, while waiting for the court to authorize involuntary treatment, the patient may continue to refuse scheduled psychiatric interventions, but emergency interventions can be provided to prevent imminent danger such as self-harm or other violence.

A court hearing to authorize or decline the involuntary treatment is conducted. In the testimony, the psychiatrist has to provide evidence that the patient has a treatable mental illness and that serious harm is likely to occur if no treatment is pursued or if it takes place in settings less restrictive than inpatient. When the court authorizes the involuntary treatment, the facility gains the legal right and the duty to administer the necessary treatment without the patient's consent. The patient loses autonomy to refuse treatment, make treatment choices, and discontinue treatment. The maximum duration of the patient's involuntary status is determined by the court, which usually grants the treating physician the option of discharging the patient before the involuntary order expires.

Medical and Legal Grounds for Coercive Interventions

There is global acceptance of the role of health care professionals in conducting interventions to prevent imminent danger when they detect such risk through a medical evaluation. The legal ground for involuntary treatment relies on widely accepted standards that as a result of a mental disorder, the patient is a danger to himself or herself, is a danger to others, or is unable to provide for his or her basic needs.

Danger to Self

The potential harm can be intentional in suicidal behaviors, unclear in serious self-inflicted injuries, and unintentional in cases of maladaptive and high-risk behaviors such as reckless driving. The danger may include harm by others in response to the patient's behaviors or direct physical or sexual assault because of failure to follow basic safety precautions. Finally, the patient's inability to follow treatment for a chronic somatic condition (e.g., dialysis for end-stage renal disease or insulin for unstable diabetes) may be a basis for unintentional harm to self.

Danger to Others

Danger to others is usually intentional and is a result of symptoms such as paranoid or persecutory delusions, command auditory hallucinations, acute intoxication, or elevated mood. Less frequently, this risk can be unintentional, such as driving recklessly and engaging in potentially dangerous behaviors (e.g., setting fires) as a result of command hallucinations. When the risk is not due to a mental health issue or is due to a condition that cannot be effectively treated in a psychiatric inpatient setting, such as impulse-control disorders or certain personality disorders, it should be addressed through legal interventions rather than involuntary admission.

Grave Disability

Grave disability is the inability to provide oneself with the basic needs of food, clothing, and shelter. For purposes of mental health law, this excludes financial incapacity. A patient not eating or drinking because of catatonia or delusions of food poisoning, exercising poor judgment as to what foods may reasonably be eaten, and not seeking shelter in dangerously cold weather are examples of failure to provide some of these essentials.

People can decline interventions for their mental health disorders as they may do for their somatic disorders. On a theoretical level, the involuntary treatment for a mental disorder does not specifically target the condition itself because people should not be involuntarily treated solely to improve their conditions. More precisely, involuntary treatment aims to mitigate the risks that can be associated with the mental disorder. Technically, these risks can be reduced either by treating the mental illness underlying these risks or by institutionalizing the patient indefinitely without treatment. Because the latter is no longer an acceptable model with the advances in mental health treatment and the global attention to human rights, involuntary treatment targeting the mental illness itself becomes the preferred way to mitigate the risks. With this understanding, the treatment cannot be forced on a patient with frank psychosis who is not in danger, but a patient with serious suicidal intent can be involuntarily hospitalized regardless of whether a mental disorder has been diagnosed.

Although suicide as a human right is controversial at the ethical level, current laws are intended to prevent most suicide and encourage medical health professionals and law enforcement authorities to intervene. Under the umbrella of law, providers have exceptional legal authority to violate the patient's rights of autonomy and confidentiality to prevent imminent harm.

Although the law does not limit the patient's autonomy to withhold life- or limb-saving treatment if he or she has the needed mental capacity to choose so, it does not allow him or her to engage in suicidal or homicidal behaviors whether he or she has the capacity to make these decisions or not and whether he or she has mental illness or not. When imminent harm is expected, the patient's mental capacity to make the decision of causing this harm is irrelevant, and interventions are launched to prevent harm based on the legal authority of the provider.

Threshold for Risk Evaluation and the Preventive Nature of Involuntary Treatment

Threats or other concerning behaviors may serve as obvious "red flags" for imminent risks. Thus, when an individual engages in threats or concerning behaviors, the community, including family members, is encouraged to inform authorities about these concerns. People may choose to call emergency hotlines or law enforcement agencies to conduct a "welfare check."

Law enforcement personnel are usually the first to respond to ensure safety and to transport the individual to the emergency department when indicated. The community effort can be counted on as a "screening test" for imminent danger with relatively high sensitivity, whereas the later evaluation by professionals in the emergency department serves as a "confirmatory test" with high specificity. In summary, the threshold to send an individual to the emergency department for evaluation of possible imminent danger is low, whereas the threshold to involuntarily admit the patient for psychiatric treatment is high and requires a professional evaluation establishing convincing evidence that imminent danger may occur unless the patient is admitted.

When the likelihood of imminent risk is deemed to be low in a patient experiencing severe or impairing symptoms, the patient is best served by voluntary inpatient treatment. There is no ground for involuntary treatment regardless of how severe the symptoms are as long as none of the involuntary commitment standards is met. When symptoms are determined to be stable or at baseline, inpatient admission is usually not indicated, and coordination of care with the outpatient provider or team is the rule.

The patient can be considered at risk for harming self or others—and hence involuntarily committable—although no actual harm has taken place yet. In fact, involuntary inpatient treatment can better serve the patient and the community when used to prevent harm rather than after it occurs. Common signs that may indicate safety concerns are verbal, media, or behavioral threats; preparatory actions such as writing notes and setting plans; and recent suicide attempts. Additionally, if certain symptoms have led to dangerous behavior in the past, similar symptoms at present may indicate the need for involuntary inpatient treatment.

Breaking the News of Involuntary Treatment

The patient's response to involuntary hospitalization may vary from apathy or sadness to extreme anger or violence. Hence, the news of involuntary admission needs to be delivered safely. Some useful tactics to evaluate the risks before you break the news are to ask the patient directly how he or she would feel if an admission were needed and to ascertain the family's expectations for the patient's possible response. A history of violence or personality disorder may increase the risk for an undesirable response. If you become concerned about possible aggression, certain arrangements should be made before news disclosure to ensure safety. The patient should be in a secure place where agitation can be contained with minimum risk, staff should be made aware, and security officers should be ready to intervene if needed. Your sincere empathy with the patient, acknowledging his or her distress and encouraging him or her to express feelings and concerns, is critical. Inquiry regarding difficulties that may result from the admission, such as childcare, work obligations, or school assignments, should be acknowledged and addressed.

In some circumstances, negotiation over legal status may be appropriate. A patient you deem too much at risk to leave the hospital may still benefit from the choice of voluntary admission. In fact, some legal venues require that patients be given this option. Although the choices do not include the freedom to leave, the patient may be able to retain other rights and avoid the stigma and loss of confidentiality of a public hearing and court order. The seeming ethical compromise of holding the threat of a court order over a patient is offset by the principles of truth-telling and maintenance of the highest level of autonomy possible.

Vignette

Dr. Z, an experienced inpatient psychiatrist, was a frequent expert witness in civil commitment cases. She appreciated the dynamic balance of ethical and legal principles involved and was careful to engage patients to the degree possible in decisions about their care. During a court hearing, she testified to having explained to her patient, Mr. B, that she had concerns about his safety after a suicide attempt and had determined that his risk was too high to leave the hospital but had given him the options of voluntary or involuntary admission. Mr. M, the patient's attorney, asked, "You didn't think it was coercive to threaten Mr. B with involuntary hospitalization if he did not agree to the treatment you recommended?" Dr. Z calmly responded, "Civil commitment is by its nature coercive; that is why we are here. He needed to know the options fully to make an informed decision. Should I have withheld information regarding the consequences of his decision to refuse voluntary treatment?" The court concurred and ordered treatment.

Ethical, Legal, and Practical Considerations

Because involuntary inpatient treatment is not planned by the patient, it often causes disruption to the patient's schedule, difficulties fulfilling obligations, and chaotic changes for the household. Patients with a history of involuntary psychiatric treatment may have difficulty obtaining some jobs, and certain legal rights like firearm ownership may be restricted. Involuntary treatment may induce feelings of powerlessness over one's health decisions or a sense of loss of control that can be frightening to some patients. With this in mind, less restrictive treatment settings should be considered first, and involuntary treatment should be pursued only when safety cannot be ensured under less restrictive treatment conditions. Indeed, the principle of "least restrictive environment" is incorporated into law in many states.

The judicial system's involvement in the final decision to mandate inpatient treatment has important benefits. First, it is consistent with the principle of direct judicial oversight of any significant restriction of rights. It is important that the decision to limit a patient's right to refuse treatment and physically leave the hospital be legal in nature and determined in an open hearing rather than being decided in a confidential team meeting by individuals solely informed by training in psychiatry. Second, the patient's presence in a formal hearing, with witness testimony and a judge's or hearing officer's ruling, may serve as a useful reality check for the patient and by itself be the basis for improved compliance with treatment. Third, it is a reality check for the treatment team, who must review the legitimacy of their observations and assertions about the case. This is particularly important when patients may make it difficult to care for them because of the strong negative emotions they may provoke. The authority given by the court for treatment should never be used to punish patients. Providers' actions must always be in the best interests of the patient. Medical judgment rather than negative countertransference should be the driving force for clinical decisions throughout the involuntary treatment. Finally, when the court authorizes involuntary treatment, the treatment dynamic may change from a power struggle between physician and patient to a view that both parties are complying with a court order that mandates treatment at this time. The perceived change in the dynamic of the relationship may make it easier to restore trust—even partially—and to reconstruct a healthier patient-physician relationship.

More often, however, involuntary treatment causes significant distress to the patient and additional strain on the therapeutic relationship. Court testimony tends to be direct, succinct, and graphic, unsoftened by euphemism or diplomacy. Patients quickly recognize that the court tends to give more credence to testimony from professionals than from patients. Because these cases are civil, rather than criminal, they are governed by a "preponderance of evidence" standard (i.e., greater than 50% certainty) rather than "beyond a reasonable doubt" (i.e., 99% certainty). Physicians are expert witnesses and therefore entitled to cite evidence that they have not personally witnessed and to express opinions. The court may even indicate that it is looking to the physician for guidance rather than just observable facts. Not surprisingly, many patients come away from these hearings angry and embittered.

Consequently, it is relatively common for patients to resist treatment in spite of a court order. Intramuscular formulations are available for only some antipsychotic and sedative agents and are not available for antidepressants or mood stabilizers. Some patients accept that they cannot avoid treatment and choose to take oral medications to facilitate discharge. Other patients who may experience improved psychotic symptoms with the forced injections become more cooperative as a result. For many, however, their compliance with treatment requires continued reason and encouragement, aided only by the knowledge that they cannot leave the hospital.

The involuntary psychiatric treatment is justified to mitigate the risk of imminent harm, and once this risk is reduced, the involuntary treatment is theoretically no longer justifiable. However, from a practical perspective and given the relapsing nature of many mental health disorders, the involuntary treatment may need to continue beyond the stabilization phase to make sure that the patient will not relapse shortly after discharge. As a result, patients should continue the involuntary treatment to allow further observation before they can safely regain autonomy—typically, after a few more days. Once the risk of imminent harm is reduced and the patient is adequately observed, treatment should continue under voluntary terms regardless of the expiration date of the authorized involuntary treatment.

Although patients have fewer rights when they are under involuntary treatment, you are ethically bound and legally mandated to attempt to accommodate their preferences if this is feasible and does not jeopardize treatment efficacy. For example, medication side effects should be addressed by changing the dose of, neutralizing, or switching the offending agent. Practically, you must work with the patient to make progress. For example, although forced treatment with antidepressant agents is legally allowed in the context of involuntary treatment, it is impractical to do so. Because of the temporary nature of the involuntary treatment, you should be aware that the best treatment for long-term benefits is the one that the patient has participated in and is able to adhere to after graduating to voluntary treatment in the community. You should carefully evaluate the need for long-acting injectable medications, the ability of the patient to follow complex dosing schedules, the ability to adhere to the needed blood work to monitor medication levels and toxicities, and the need for involuntary outpatient treatment to ensure adherence depending on the expected risks for future relapses.

Competency and Consent

Competency refers to individuals' ability to make decisions for themselves. Although this term is widely used in medical practice, it is a legal rather than a medical concept, referring to decision-making capacity over personal, financial, legal, and medical issues. Competency may be affected, however, by psychiatric and other medical conditions; thus, your role as a psychiatrist is critical in assessing those capacities. Competency is not an "all-or-nothing" concept but rather is relative to specific tasks and issues. Thus, a patient may be capable of deciding to accept antacid for heartburn but not to consent to a kidney donation.

Informed consent in health care is a process by which knowledge about a medical issue and proposed intervention is communicated from experts to patients to help them make decisions about their health. Hence, this is a two-way process because it requires education by the clinician and understanding by the patient before a decision can be made. This process—called the informed consent—should be completed before any medical intervention such as prescription of a medication or performance of a procedure.

Medical Consent for Treatment

The process of the informed consent is a legal and ethical responsibility for you as the provider and a right for your patient. The process involves explanation of the elements of the consent and opportunities for the patient to ask questions. The patient makes a decision based on the information provided and the patient's preferences. With substantial decisions, such as for major procedures, the process usually involves written and verbal consent. Informed consent, however, is a process and not just a signature and should be "conducted" and not just "obtained."

Elements of Informed Consent

You should disclose all information that is pertinent to the proposed intervention during the consent process. Use language that is appropriate for the knowledge level of the individual patient, with a minimum of technical jargon. In general, the following issues are sufficient to establish informed consent for most medical interventions.

Main Problem, Illness, or Symptoms

Give a simple and general description of the illness for which the intervention is proposed. Information may be provided about the illness nature, main characteristics, related symptoms, prognosis, and other relevant issues.

Proposed Intervention

Introduce the patient to the intervention with a nontechnical description of its specific aspects and the steps by which it is done.

Intervention-Related Benefits

Describe the possible positive outcomes of the intervention, such as experiencing partial or full alleviation of symptoms, slowing or blocking further deterioration, preventing complications, and improving prognosis, as well as indirect benefits such as maintaining independence and improving ability to function.

Intervention-Related Risks or Complications

Include short- and long-term medication side effects or procedure complications. Numerous negative outcomes are possible, and although informed consent is not expected to cover all that is in the literature, try to summarize the most common and serious ones. Special attention should be made to address risks that are more relevant to the individual patient, such as weight gain for a patient with obesity, other cardiovascular risk factors, or teratogenicity risk for a woman of childbearing age.

Alternative Interventions

Give a brief description of interventions other than the proposed one and how they may serve the patient comparatively. Include why these alternatives are considered equivalent, second line, less optimal, or not advised. Always discuss the option of no intervention, with its possible consequences.

The five elements of informed consent (illness, intervention, benefits, risks, alternatives) can be remembered by the mnemonic "I Identify Benefits and Risks for All my patients." The use of this phrase is especially helpful for trainees, but even experienced practitioners may benefit from occasional reminders.

Informed Consent in Inpatient Psychiatric Treatment

Informed consent should precede any intervention for the voluntarily hospitalized patient but is not required for those receiving involuntary treatment. Patients with guardians cannot give consent, and their guardians must give consent on their behalf.

Involuntary patients retain the right to be treated respectfully in line with the ethical principle of justice. They should be informed about treatments and given opportunities to ask questions, but their approval is not required. Practically, educating patients undergoing involuntary treatment or those who are not their own guardians about the intervention and having them participate by asking questions and even by choosing treatment options, if possible, may build a better therapeutic alliance and encourage them to cooperate with treatment.

The ability of patients to understand issues relevant to their illnesses and proposed interventions varies greatly. For patients with limited cognitive ability, thought disorganization, or delusions regarding treatment, basic understanding is all that is needed for their consent. For example, establishing that patients with psychosis understand that they are offered antipsychotic agents because they have an illness and to "stop the voices" would be adequate. It is critical, however, that there be no deception, such as telling a patient that an antipsychotic is just to help with sleep or a mood stabilizer is to prevent a seizure. The greater problem with these patients is their ability to understand major side effects and to maintain their commitment to treatment, both of which require specific discussion.

Most adults are assumed to be competent unless a legal determination indicates that they are not. Hence, there is no need to prove that an adult has capacity to make general medical decisions. Mental health patients, by contrast, are often assumed by medical teams, family members, and lawmakers not to be competent. Such individuals' competency may be questioned because of intellectual disability, active psychotic symptoms, extreme mood states, or a pattern of poor decisions. Your job as a psychiatric consultant is to sort through which symptoms affect competency to make specific decisions and which do not.

Guardianship

For the individual who is unable to process information, rationally make choices, or articulate a basis for decisions, surrogate decision-making is the preferred option. Concerns about a patient's capacity often will be expressed by the medical team or family members. Occasionally, the issue may be raised by Child or Adult Protective Services, community mental health agencies, or law enforcement authorities. When confirmed by a formal competency assessment, additional steps must take place to establish who will be empowered to make decisions on behalf of the patient. One option is for the family, public agencies, or the medical center to petition the court to appoint a guardian.

A court appointed guardian, who can be a family member, has the duty to make decisions that are objectively in the best interest of the individual, even if they do not reflect the incompetent individual's wishes or are even against them. The designated guardian makes decisions for the incompetent individual at all times regardless of the individual's mental state, and this authority remains in effect until it is revoked by the court.

Appointment of a guardian is a substantial decision that curtails rights of freedom and autonomy. The legal threshold is high and requires abundant evidence of impairment leading to medical relapses, legal consequences, or inability to function independently. The process typically takes weeks to months, even when it is not contested. If the patient is opposed or there is a disagreement over who should serve as guardian, it may take longer. In acute situations, such as a life-threatening injury or illness, temporary authorization—emergency guardianship—can be obtained within a few days.

Civil commitment and the appointment of a guardian are separate legal processes that address different issues and are not equivalent to each other. Civil commitment is about a need for treatment to maintain safety and does not imply incapacity to make other decisions. Guardianship is about lack of competence to make decisions but does not include the legal right to force an individual to accept treatment. This is a critical distinction that plays out frequently in hospital settings.

Legally, incompetent individuals cannot consent to treatment, and their guardians provide consent on their behalf for all care, including admission, medication management, medical procedures, and disposition planning (with limitations regarding electroconvulsive therapy in some states). Although the patient's consent is not legally required, it is more ethical and practical to involve the patient in making decisions for himself or herself whenever this is feasible. More important, if the patient refuses to cooperate with treatment, a guardian cannot force him or her to comply, and a separate civil commitment process may be necessary to authorize involuntary treatment.

Advance Directives, Living Wills, and Durable Powers of Attorney for Health Care

In the absence of the patient's ability to consent for treatment, several alternatives to guide medical decisions exist. In anticipation of such situations, people may choose—in advance—to designate a surrogate decision-maker through a living will (i.e., a will that becomes active while the patient is still living), advance directive, or durable power of attorney for health care (i.e., authority to make decisions that remains in effect even when the person granting the authority is incapacitated). Most of these were designed for general medical care rather than mental health issues and are more appropriate for patients who have just had a cardiac arrest or are in a coma than for those whose capacity to make decisions is affected by altered thought processes or extreme mood states. In fact, only a few venues recognize them as legally binding in psychiatric conditions, and the process of determining whether someone's mental status qualifies as debilitating is usually similar, if not identical, to that used for appointment of a guardian.

This may be a point of contention with family members, who incorrectly believe that being designated as a surrogate decision-maker grants them authority to direct treatment. In these cases, your understanding of these legal processes will be essential to confidently directing treatment and engaging the family in a discussion of the limits of these documents. If questions persist, consultation with the hospital attorney is a useful next step.

Advance directives may serve a useful function for individuals at high risk for recurrent involuntary hospitalization, such as those with schizophrenia or bipolar disorder. In these cases, patients may express preferences for specific medications, contact with certain individuals, or treatment in designated facilities. Although not legally binding, these preferences may be useful to the treatment team in making decisions about the patient's care when he or she is acutely agitated, markedly delusional, catatonic, oppositional, or otherwise unable to participate in treatment planning.

Confidentiality

You have a duty to keep patients' personal data private and not release it to a third party without their consent. This concept is considered one of the ethical standards for many professions, such as medicine, law, banking, and education. Within medicine, the Health Insurance Portability and Accountability Act (HIPAA) is the current federal legislation that regulates confidentiality in the United States. All data containing personal or clinical information about the patient are classified as protected health information and hence are bound by confidentiality regulations. This includes but is not limited to the patient's name, date of birth, telephone number, address, medical record number, and clinical data, as well as the fact that the patient is under the care of a provider or a facility.

Parents or legal guardians of a minor patient may be exceptions to the confidentiality regulations because their knowledge of the patient's condition is essential in making decisions for their child. Certain adolescent health issues, however, such as substance abuse, sexually transmitted diseases and their treatment, and contraception services, may be subject to confidentiality regulations, and their parents or legal guardians do not always have the right to access this information. Legal venues differ significantly regarding a child's rights to privacy and the ages at which those rights may change. Be aware of the laws that apply where you are practicing to avoid any potential problems.

To comply with the federal and state regulations, medical facilities maintain internal policies to prevent unauthorized data sharing. For example, most hospitals require a specific form to be signed by the patient to release his or her records to a third party, but they also may require written permission for you to speak with employers, friends, and even family members. Discussion of patients' information is prohibited in public areas such as hallways, cafeterias, elevators, and waiting rooms. Paper charts are kept private, and access to the electronic medical records is regulated through passwords. Periodically, staff are required to complete certain trainings to ensure being up to date with the confidentiality policies, procedures, and precautions.

Confidentiality and Mental Health

The privacy of mental health information may be even more important for patients than other medical health information. Various reasons may underlie the desire to keep this information private such as shame, denial, and fear of stigma. The history of psychotic illness, substance use disorder, treatment with psychotropic medications, and involuntary treatment may be barriers to certain jobs or to legally own firearms.

Consequently, mental health information may have extra protection beyond that applied to general medical records. This may include authorization to enter specific portions of an electronic medical record, separate records for general medical and mental health care, and an electronic "firewall" that allows only mental health professionals to gain access to or even see the date of a psychiatric record. Psychotherapists may choose to omit from notes private and exceptionally sensitive information that has no specific medical implications. The wisdom and efficacy of these measures are highly debatable, but you should be aware of the procedures where you work to ensure your compliance with them.

Breaking Confidentiality

Medical health information is confidential by default, but in some situations, confidentiality may, and in a few cases must, be violated. Many of the most common scenarios in which information may be provided regardless of the patient's consent occur during hospital-based psychiatric care.

Emergency Situations

In emergency situations, the patient may not be able to consent for various reasons, such as loss of consciousness, severe distress, or intense behavioral dyscontrol. If the patient's medical record is deemed essential to save the patient's life, consent to release information is not required, and the facility, the agency, or the provider contacted for these records or information is excused from obtaining formal consent to release this information. Because many patients use the emergency department as an urgent care unit, the emergency exception to confidentiality should be used only in truly life-threatening situations, and the patient's presence in the emergency department is not adequate justification to break confidentiality. The information requested or shared should be limited to what is necessary to handle the critical condition, and attempts should be made to obtain the consent of the patient as soon as the situation allows.

Imminent Risk to Harm Oneself

Assessment of suicide risk is a fundamental component of every psychiatric examination. Many patients, either before or after engaging in self-harm, deny or refuse to discuss their actions. Collateral information is essential to your assessment of the patient's likelihood of engaging in suicidal behavior after leaving your care. Both ethical standards and legal regulations permit confidentiality to be breached in these cases, allowing you to contact whomever you feel is best equipped to share critical information. Most commonly, this will include family, close friends, and current or recent care providers.

Imminent Risk to Harm Others

You must break confidentiality if necessary to prevent harm to another individual. *Tarasoff* laws, originally intended to protect mental health professionals who choose to violate confidentiality to protect a patient or someone from a patient, have gradually evolved into a positive requirement to act in these situations. In most cases in which a patient poses a threat because of a psychiatric disorder, involuntary admission is appropriate. In some cases, however, other action may be required. Most often, this will include contact with the intended victim and disclosure of the threat to law enforcement authorities.

Child Abuse

If a patient discloses past or ongoing abuse, including physical and sexual abuse or neglect, or intention for future abuse of a child, Child Protective Services must be notified to investigate the situation and intervene to protect the child if needed. Confidentiality must be broken even if the perpetrator is not the identified patient or when this report is provided by people other than the patient. When imminent danger to a child is expected, the potential perpetrator should be detained until the child is placed in safe custody. The threshold for breaking confidentiality in these situations is low, and even a suspicion of abuse justifies and mandates reporting it. Because this threshold is low and clinicians are mandatory reporters, you are legally protected from potential lawsuits or other legal actions.

Elder Abuse and the Abuse of Vulnerable Adults

The same regulations and steps taken to protect children from abuse are followed to protect older patients and other adults with mental or physical disabilities rendering them vulnerable to abuse. In these situations, Adult Protective Services must be notified to investigate the situation and to make interventions to ensure the safety of older or vulnerable adults.

Court Reports and Testimony

In cases of civil commitment, guardianship appointment, child custody, testamentary capacity, disability claims, competency to stand trial, and assessment of criminal responsibility, you may be called on to provide expert testimony to the court. Court proceedings are generally open to the public, and records or written reports submitted to the court become public documents, so confidentiality is not maintained in these cases. Your expert opinion may play a substantial role in these proceedings, making it unethical to withhold information from the court because of confidentiality concerns. To avoid this pitfall, you have a duty to inform the individual—in advance—of the specific nature of these evaluations and that confidentiality will not be maintained.

This should be self-evident when your involvement in the case is solely for forensic purposes, but it also applies to cases in which your primary responsibility to the patient is clinical, such as an emergency department evaluation that may result in involuntary treatment. You should warn patients about this exception to the usual standards of confidentiality as soon as you realize that civil commitment is a possibility, even if it complicates your relationship with the patient and makes information more difficult to obtain. Intentional deception, including by omission of information, is a poor therapeutic intervention even when done with the best of intentions.

Limitations to Rights of Privacy and Autonomy

Behavioral volatility may carry risks of serious physical injury in emergency, psychiatric, and general medical units. Risks include elopement, agitation, self-injurious behavior, suicide, and aggression. Targets for these behaviors can be property, the patient, other patients, visitors, and staff. On inpatient psychiatric units, these risks are of particular importance and are one of the topics discussed daily by the treatment team. Safety is maintained through routine general precautions and specific interventions to address emergency situations, each of which involves some abrogation of individual rights.

Safety Precautions and Limits of Privacy

To ensure safety, general precautions are maintained throughout all phases of hospital care. Most inpatient psychiatric units are locked, and patients may not leave without adequate evaluation. At entry, every patient and visitor should be screened for weapons and other dangerous objects. Access to personal clothing, although an internationally recognized right of mental health patients, may be limited by safety concerns, with restrictions on items such as belts, scarves, and shoelaces. Patients using medical equipment such as canes, feeding tubes, needles for self-administered medications, and sleep apnea devices must be closely monitored, and use of such equipment may require direct supervision.

Safety checks, in which a staff member directly observes each patient, are maintained throughout the admission at intervals ranging from every 30 minutes to continuous observation based on the individual patient's level of risk. These checks must be frequent enough to allow early detection of potentially dangerous behavior and rapid intervention if it occurs. Privacy concerns sometimes may be sacrificed, and doors of patients' rooms and bathrooms are not lockable, to allow observation and emergency intervention.

Security cameras may be appropriate in some areas, especially emergency settings, inpatient hallways and community areas, and seclusion rooms. Patients should be notified of these cameras, the locations that are and are not monitored, and whether a video recording is made. Use of security cameras is generally a backup system and should not take the place of direct observation by staff. None of these safety procedures is considered extraordinarily invasive, and none requires specific documentation or review.

Restraint of Free Movement

Restraint refers to the coercive restriction of a patient's free movement beyond that required to prevent elopement from the facility. Staff physically holding any part of a patient's body; locking the patient in a confined space that lacks the full facilities of a hospital inpatient unit; or placing bonds on body, head, or limbs all constitute forms of restraint. Accepted uses of restraint include to stop ongoing harm (e.g., head banging), to prevent imminent harm (e.g., threatened assault), and to compel compliance with court-ordered treatment (e.g., medication administration). Interventions that patients request or voluntarily accept to help calm themselves down or avoid violence, such as taking a sedative medication or isolating themselves in a quiet room, are not considered forms of restraint. Similarly, consented restraint, such as that done during medical transport, surgery, or electroconvulsive therapy, is not coercive in nature and does not require the same procedures as involuntary restraint.

No form of restraint is permissible unless other less restrictive measures have failed or been deemed inadequate, and the form of restraint used must be the least restrictive possible. Based on extensive discussion with patients and patient-rights groups, verbal de-escalation is considered least invasive, followed by voluntary medication, involuntary medication, room seclusion, and finally four-point restraints.

All forms of involuntary restraint require specific documentation of the basis for the action, the action taken, and the time involved. This level of documentation is intended to ensure that these actions are not done arbitrarily or punitively, but are therapeutically necessary to maintain safety. Restraints should not be used to address other patient issues, such as being rude, disrespectful, demanding, or otherwise annoying to staff. Various state and professional organizations (e.g., The Joint Commission) exercise oversight, reviewing both individual cases and larger institutional patterns of patient restraint, with the goal of limiting its use to the minimum possible number of cases while ensuring the safety of patients and staff.

Seclusion or Environmental Restraint

Seclusion is the least restrictive form of restraint, which involves confinement of the patient in a restricted space, usually a single room designated for safety. The purpose is to minimize stimulation and allow the patient to calm down without taking more aggressive measures. Seclusion may be performed in the patient's room in the inpatient unit, whereas more dramatic situations may require placing the patient in a designated room—a seclusion or quiet room—with continuous monitoring. This form of restraint is appropriate when the patient is engaging in or threatening aggressive behaviors toward others but is not actively doing things that are harmful to self. It also may be applied to minimize unit disruption caused by patient behaviors such as screaming and marked agitation.

Therapeutic or Physical Hold

Any physical contact with a patient by a staff member that is intended to exercise control of the patient is a form of restraint. Thus, a nurse taking the arm of an ataxic patient to help maintain balance would not be restraint but holding that same patient's arm while an involuntary medication is injected would be. Most such restraint is brief and occurs as other interventions are being provided. For example, physical management of the patient may be needed to place the patient in seclusion when resistance occurs. The physical hold is likewise an integral part in the process of applying restraint devices.

Restraint Devices

This is the most aggressive and restrictive type of restraint, in which the patient's ability to move is restricted by bands most often applied to wrists and ankles (four-point restraint) and occasionally other parts of the body such as the torso. Bands are typically made of leather, cloth, or plastic; metal restraints are limited to criminal law enforcement and are not permissible in mental health settings. Because of its highly confining nature, this procedure is usually the last resort after other less restrictive measures fail to ensure safety.

Process of Restraint Administration

Restraint administration can be physically and emotionally exhausting for both patients and staff. Training is key to make this intervention efficient, effective, harmless, and less traumatizing. While applying restraints, certain issues must be considered.

First, your decision to use any form of restraint should be based on medical necessity rather than convenience or an emotional reaction to the patient. You may take the patient's expressed preference in an advance directive or during the event into consideration but should never compromise safety in doing so.

Second, patients may resist the attempt to apply restraint, which may predispose them to physical injuries. Hence, a physical examination should follow any rough physical contact with the patient. Any physical injury should be handled appropriately. A physical examination also may be necessary after the use of sedative medications to check for dystonic reactions or unstable vital signs. Observation and management of injuries should continue to the degree possible, even as patients attempt to escape or fight restraints.

Third, it is not uncommon for the patient to become more aggressive while restraints are being applied and intentionally or unintentionally cause injury to the staff involved. Although staff are encouraged to protect themselves in the process, they are only allowed to act defensively and may not take offensive action such as striking the patient. The presence of an adequate number of staff and appropriate training in the procedure are essential.

Fourth, effort should be made to preserve the patient's dignity insofar as is possible. Try to explain the procedure and the need for it to the patient before applying it, or when this is not feasible because of rapid escalation in behavior, take the time after restraint administration to educate the patient about it (e.g., why, how, for how long). Possible complications such as physical injuries and medication side effects also should be explained. Patients should be allowed to ask questions and to express feelings and concerns. They also should be encouraged to bring issues for medical attention such as unseen physical injuries.

Finally, limits are placed on how long an order for restraint may be continued, typically 4 hours for adults and 2 hours for children; whether it can be renewed; and what level of evaluation must be conducted for it to be renewed. In all cases, it should be continued only for the minimum time consistent with safety.

KEY POINTS

- Mental health law, in contrast to laws governing other health care, generally assumes that patients may not be able to act autonomously and may even need protection, that patients usually do not want and must specifically request mental health care, and that many aspects of this care require intense legal scrutiny.

- When major safety concerns arise, the psychiatrist has legal authority to detain a patient for evaluation and may seek court-ordered treatment.

- The legal ground for involuntary treatment includes the diagnosis of a mental disorder leading to a danger to oneself, a danger to others, or an inability to provide for one's basic needs.

- Adults with mental health issues are competent unless a court decides that they are not. Legal guardians make decisions for incompetent individuals.

- Informed consent should precede any voluntary treatment. Consent is not required for involuntary treatment, but in most cases, the patient should be fully informed.

- The five elements of informed consent (illness, intervention, benefits, risks, alternatives) can be remembered by the mnemonic, "I Identify Benefits and Risks for All my patients."

- Medical health information is confidential, and specific authorization from the patient is required before information may be shared, except in life-threatening emergencies, including emergency department suicide assessments.

- Restraint procedures are applied to stop current harm, prevent impending harm, or comply with court-ordered treatment. In these cases, the principle of least restrictive treatment always should be followed.

CHAPTER 15

Quality Assessment and Improvement

Nasuh Malas, M.D., M.P.H.

In the age of managed care,
payers have increasingly focused on health care quality, population health, and cost reduction, while increasing patient choices in their care. Consumers seek high-quality services that are efficient, have a relatively low cost, and produce consistent, positive outcomes. Greater focus in hospital settings on the development of clinical pathways, protocols, and guidelines has spurred quality measurement. These quality measures may serve to reinforce your use of practice guidelines and policies, often attached to certain consequences or incentives.

The Medicare Access and CHIP (Children's Health Insurance Program) Reauthorization Act of 2015 (P.L. 114-10) has clear language prioritizing quality assessment and improvement with an emphasis on value-based payment and incentives for quality care. The Centers for Medicare and Medicaid Services, the National Committee for Quality Assurance, and The Joint Commission monitor, report, and incentivize quality assurance measures. These measures are increasingly being required for reporting as comparators between care settings and as sources for incentivizing care. For example, as a provider participating in the Medicare meaningful use incentive program, you are required to report on a set of clinical quality measures as outlined by the U.S. National Quality Strategy. Other Medicare-based programs reward you for meeting certain outlined clinical quality standards.

In 2006, the Institute of Medicine Committee found that the infrastructure, resources, and ability to address quality in psychiatric care were significantly underdeveloped with little communication between mental health, substance use, and physical health services. Mental health is ripe for quality assessment and quality improvement yet has lagged other specialty areas. The lack of quality assessment and improvement is likely related to challenges in practice variability, limited validated metrics, and minimal study in quality. Given the rapidly changing landscape in inpatient mental health care, you must be equipped to understand and apply quality assurance measures, while adjusting practice based on the input gathered from those measures.

Unfortunately, inpatient psychiatry is at a relative disadvantage with limited tools to demonstrate value and quality of care. The National Quality Forum, a nonprofit public-private joint endeavor focused on improving health care quality in the United States, has identified more than 700 measures in health care aimed at quality assessment, but only 30 of these measures are directly related to mental health service. Of the 33 quality measures provided by the Centers for Medicare and Medicaid Services, only one measure—depression screening and follow-up—relates to psychiatric care.

In this environment of limited availability of quality measures, mental health providers face a challenge to demonstrate the efficacy of what we do. Consequently, funding is diverted from mental health to other areas of health care that can show quality improvement and value. The end result is high variability, lack of transparency, lack of incentives for higher-quality care, and missed opportunities to empower mental health systems to engage in quality improvement efforts.

Quality Assessment and Measurement

Assessment of quality is focused on the functional outcome of the process of giving and receiving care. Functional outcomes are influenced by changes in the disease course with improvement or resolution. Ultimately, these actions are predicated on resources, staffing, and environmental structures needed to provide care.

Along the continuum from inputs to functional outcomes are opportunities to assess, develop, and report on quality. These measures can be used to enhance care quality or support patients' understanding about the quality of care they are receiving. Measures can serve to compare the quality of services within a larger system to assess high and low performing areas. Quality measures can be instrumental to ensure that a minimum standard is maintained. Payers access quality measures to aid in assessing service value and differential reimbursement of services.

Determining what to measure, how to measure, and at what level you intend to measure a given aspect of psychiatric care can be fraught with challenges. Psychiatric care measures are naturally more abstract and less measurable than other health-related quality measures. It can be difficult to develop measures that answer the specific question or questions identified and to determine whether that measure is sustainable and provides meaningful data over time.

The focus of quality assessment in inpatient psychiatric care settings has been on input and process measures. Progress has been spurred predominantly by payers looking to enhance performance. Input and process measures are often preferred by payers to incentivize certain aspects of care because they are easily measurable and can limit selection biases, while giving the provider a sense of influence and control in addressing a given measure. These often include measures of access, utilization, and care provision (such as use of antidepressants or antipsychotics for a given indication), as well as monitoring of clinical responses to treatment over time with standardized rating scales. These metrics, particularly if narrowly defined, can be easily attained from regularly collected clinical or administrative data, reducing the cost and disruptions involved in obtaining data. However, these measures also may result in providers or systems changing behavior to meet the specific standard, while detracting the focus from comprehensive quality care.

This approach can devalue the true effect of psychiatric care on clinical and functional outcomes, failing to recognize the importance of issues such as patients' experience of care, changes in the disease process, enhancements in quality of life or functioning, and the effect on cost. Input and process measures do not fully capture the necessary quality metrics to highlight the importance of mental health care and assess factors such as access to care, screening, and receipt of evidence-based care for a given condition. This approach does not account for the value created by the downstream effects on patient care. The relative lack of clinical and functional outcomes represents one of the biggest gaps in quality assessment in psychiatric care.

Functional outcome measures have the powerful potential to highlight the value of mental health evaluation and treatment to patients, health sys-

tems, schools, employers, payers, and the community. It is important to select an adequate and diverse array of functional outcomes, so that several
measures of how patients are doing in real life can be grouped together
rather than focusing on individual, isolated items. Metrics include patients'
workplace productivity; ability to sustain employment; and effects on work
absenteeism, living arrangements, functionality, substance use, legal involvement, and overall health. Use of technologies has been increasing to
obtain functional outcome data, which was found to be acceptable and
achievable for collecting patient-reported assessments of psychiatric care.
Increasing evidence indicates that patient-reported functional outcome
measures can be incorporated into routine psychiatric care and result in
tangible quality improvements. Table 15–1 outlines the types of quality
measures involved in each stage of this process, beginning with an evaluation of resources (inputs), assessment of clinical processes, and monitoring
of changes in clinical processes with specific interventions (outputs) and
ending with measures of patients' level of recovery and functional capacity.

Goals and Considerations in Quality Assessment

We identify several factors in Table 15–2 for you to consider in selecting
and assessing quality measures for use in practice.

Feasibility and Psychometric Properties

Any measure you select needs to be assessed for interrater reliability, validity, psychometric properties, and overall statistical strength as a quality
measure. This is often assessed in concert with a statistician and with input
from those using and measuring the given quality metric. Furthermore,
your ability to operationalize the use and reporting of the measure, cost
considerations, feasibility of longitudinal data collection, and analysis of the
added value of using a given measure must be assessed before implementation. In general, simple, straightforward, low-cost measures that are easy to
collect, fit well within usual workflow, and have strong psychometric properties have the highest yield in quality assessment and improvement.

Transparency

Quality measures create an environment of transparency for consumers,
fostering greater opportunity for quality improvement. Transparency in-
stills greater confidence in those receiving, providing, or funding care. It

TABLE 15–1. Continuum of quality measurement from inputs to functional outcomes

Input measures	These quantify whether a given setting has the resources, structures, and staffing to provide high-quality care for given symptoms or conditions.
	Resources and environment should match patient needs and evidence-based standards.
	Example: Presence of clinicians trained in family-based interventions within an inpatient eating disorder program.
Process measures	These assess interventions used to provide patient care and degree to which that care meets current evidence-based standards.
	They capture transitions in care, care integration, communication across settings, and care coordination.
	Measures can span beyond direct care implementation and include actions facilitating care, such as calling a place of employment or speaking to the patient's primary care physician.
	Example: Application of cognitive-behavioral therapy for a patient with generalized anxiety disorder.
Clinical output measures	These are generated from care processes or services provided to meet patient care needs.
	They can assess effect of care on disease or on patient knowledge and skills that can promote future symptomatic improvement.
	Example: Monitoring improvement in patient-reported depression scale scores over time while treating the patient with psychotherapy and a selective serotonin reuptake inhibitor.
Functional output measures	These assess improvement in functionality, quality of life, or definable change in health or behavior.
	They are the end result in patient's care if all previous steps in the process generate anticipated results.
	These measures match specific expectations of disease presentation and course in a given population.
	Example: Ability to maintain meaningful employment or continued housing in a patient with schizophrenia.

TABLE 15–2. Considerations in selection of quality measurement

Feasibility

Psychometric properties

Transparency

Accountability

Differential emphasis

Perceived provider influence

Patient selectivity

Scope of focus

enhances collaborative decision-making to increase efficiency and quality of care. Clinical and functional outcomes tend to support transparency to a greater extent than input and process measures do. Even if patients pay little attention to reported quality measures, these measures can still have a significant effect on quality by allowing providers or payers to observe, compare, and reflect on their own performance, both over time and among their peers.

Accountability

Performance that is measured, reported, and incentivized creates a sense of accountability to provide quality care. Whether to promote minimum standards of care, or drive providers to higher-quality care, quality measures can significantly affect provider behaviors. The direct motivation for providers is to meet or exceed quality standards through monetary or other performance incentives. There is also the psychological benefit to providers whose professionalism leads them to perform their duties to the best of their abilities. This inherently creates a culture focused on constant quality assessment and improvement.

Provider practice is more likely to change if performance feedback is longitudinal, regular, and coupled closely with meaningful incentives. Quality measures should be designed with anticipation of how the act of reporting will affect behavior, with attention to the potential positive and negative consequences on provider behavior, perception, and care.

Differential Emphasis

Quality measures inherently place a greater value on certain care practices, structures, or outcomes based on which aspects of care are emphasized. This creates important considerations in selecting measures that may result in a differential emphasis on certain aspects of care. Addressing one quality standard may negatively affect another aspect of care, measured or not. For example, high patient satisfaction may not necessarily translate into improved functional outcomes. This can cause an overly focused approach to some aspects of care at the expense of others, with deleterious consequences. Therefore, it is important for you to balance the need to focus on quality in certain areas without reducing the overall quality of care.

Perceived Provider Influence

You may feel limited ability to influence measured outcomes. Psychosocial, cultural, and inherent patient-related factors may make you perceive that you cannot have a tangible effect on a given quality measure. You may also perceive that such measures do not affect overall care quality. You may believe that the data and assumptions used to develop a measure are inaccurate. Factors such as time, cost, training, workflow, and personal belief about quality of care can also affect your willingness to engage in a quality measure.

A mismatch between a quality measure and your perceived influence on that measure can generate a negative attitude toward the measure. This can be counterproductive, making it imperative to assess the effect of your perception on a quality measure and how that measure is used. Even if your perceived influence is low, the measure may still be helpful for certain stakeholders, such as patients, to improve informed decision-making. For example, knowledge of your proficiency in certain aspects of psychotherapy will be helpful to patients selecting a provider who aligns with their care needs.

Patient Selectivity

Depending on the quality measures selected, you may have a conscious or unconscious bias toward certain "desirable" patients. This is similar to differential emphasis, whereby selection of a quality measure may have other systemic unintended negative consequences on service provision, allocation, and provider behavior. You may be tempted to provide care for patients who more easily allow for meeting or exceeding quality standards but dissuade patients deemed more "challenging" or "difficult." Establishment of broader population measures rather than a focus on small subgroups or narrowly defined measures based on specific patient qualities can mitigate this issue.

Scope of Focus

It is critical to determine whether the selected quality assessment is narrow or broad. Narrow measures allow for more concrete, clear, and measurable targets. These focused data can raise the standard of care to an accepted evidence-based approach or consensus standard by providing a well-defined outline of how or what care should be offered. However, narrow measures can, at times, limit innovation, flexibility, and adaptability. Broader assessments may promote more creativity and empower providers or systems with natural incentives to explore novel approaches to care.

Application of Quality Measurement

Involuntary Admission

Psychoeducation and crisis avoidance measures can be helpful in inpatient psychiatry, highlighted in the involuntary admission process. At times, involuntary admission is necessary and permissible to ensure the safety of a patient who may pose a danger to self or others because of psychiatric illness. However, involuntary admission can significantly affect the patient's personal investment in the admission, diminishing the potential therapeutic effect of the inpatient stay with increased risk of negative consequences. Therefore, prevention of involuntary admission can have far-reaching effects.

Several strategies have been found to be effective in stemming involuntary admission. One approach involves the development of a joint crisis plan between the patient, a care coordinator, and the treating psychiatrist. The use of a patient-centered preventive crisis plan has resulted in a significant reduction in involuntary admissions and days of involuntary commitment and has been found to be highly cost-effective. The underlying premise is that psychoeducation focused on patient risk factors for crisis development, as well as close monitoring to detect early signs of crisis, can provide early opportunities to stem escalation of disease and behaviors, thus preventing crises that may result in involuntary admission. Another approach is the use of crisis cards or documents that can be carried by the patient that specify critical diagnostic and treatment information, key contacts, potential triggers for crisis, and strategies that have worked for the patient to allow for de-escalation. These interventions can be coupled to provide a comprehensive preventive approach, including individualized psychoeducation, close collaboration with the patient to identify antecedent triggers and calming strategies for illness-related crisis, use of customized crisis tools, and preventive monitoring of high-risk individuals or specific risk factors.

Patient Satisfaction

Consumer trust in the mental health system strongly predicts the perception of the quality of inpatient mental health care. The reverse is also true, and the perceived quality of the inpatient experience predicts degree of trust in mental health care. Some studies have found that improved patient satisfaction following inpatient psychiatric care is a proxy for high-quality processes during the stay. This perception is often so powerful that it generalizes beyond the inpatient stay to the larger mental health system. Patient satisfaction surveys have an inherent bias because the patients who complete satisfaction surveys often give favorable ratings to their providers. This factor has dissuaded some systems from use of patient-reported satisfaction surveys. However, if the surveys are structured to assess multiple dimensions, these assessments can be highly valuable tools to distinguish quality among settings and providers.

Hospital Readmission

Readmission rates are one of the most widely used quality measures in inpatient psychiatry, serving as a proxy for relapse, failure of care after discharge, or inadequate care within the hospital setting. Readmission meets many of the criteria for a valuable quality measure, including feasibility, ease of reporting, and importance, because rehospitalization rates can easily be collected from administrative records with good quality and reliability. Measurement of readmission should be proximal to discharge but allow enough time for appropriate follow-up and activation of community supports. Readmission rates should take into account the acuity, severity, and nature of the underlying psychiatric conditions.

Discharge readiness is key to reducing readmission, including early prescription of appropriate medications and doses, acceptance and establishment of prompt outpatient follow-up, and increase in family involvement. Timely follow-up after hospitalization can reduce the duration of disability and the likelihood of rehospitalization and is an important quality indicator relating to readmission. Patient satisfaction with care and therapeutic alliance with the inpatient treatment team do not appear to be correlated to readmission rates.

Numerous other factors also have an effect on readmission rate, both inside and outside your control. Among these are patient-specific factors such as previous hospitalization, severity of mental illness (particularly presence of psychosis, self-injurious behavior, thought disorganization, and agitation), substance use, poor treatment adherence, and younger age. Social factors include previous incarceration, lack of meaningful employment, inadequate social supports, unstable living environment, and lack of access to transportation. Systems-level risk factors include the quality and avail-ability of community-based psychiatric care and insurance coverage.

Readmission rates have been challenging to address because of a lack of clinical data to capture all the factors involved and steps taken to address them. Symptom severity is the usual focus of inpatient care. Comorbid substance use may be addressed during admission or through intensive, evidence-based, community-based, dual-diagnosis care in the community. Improvements in housing, income, and employment are difficult during hospitalization, but effective social work interventions can ameliorate some of these issues. Careful discharge planning with attention to prompt follow-up will further reduce risk. Thus, readmission rate is a strong indicator of the overall effectiveness of treatment but is less useful in targeting specific deficiencies in care.

Seclusion and Restraint

Seclusion and restraint use is an important safety metric in the inpatient setting. Several approaches have been successful in limiting these invasive interventions, including institutional policies, specialized training programs, psychoeducation, patient education in self-management strategies, greater self-awareness among staff, and interpersonal conflict management. A review of restraint history and medication preferences may help you develop a crisis management program that includes identification of potential triggers and calming strategies for behavioral escalation. Staff training may include symptom recognition, agitation rating scales, verbal interventions, behavior plans, and use of as-needed medication. One effective strategy is to create a crisis management plan for each high-acuity patient, including factors that may precipitate crisis and therapeutic de-escalation strategies, which you review each week with your care team. At the moment of escalation, the patient's crisis plan is employed, after which you conduct a focused debriefing to review what went well and what needed improvement.

Medication Safety

The secure and safe reconciliation, prescription, and dissemination of medications from admission to discharge is a critical aspect of care within the hospital setting. Medication errors are reported at rates of 2%–15% in both medical and psychiatric inpatient settings. Most studies, however, gather information on medication errors and adverse drug events by self-report, which grossly underrepresents these medication safety metrics when compared with careful review of the medical record.

Errors in prescription and administration are most common, usually as a result of omission of prescribed medications on admission or at discharge; missing prescription information; or incorrect prescription dose, frequency, or formulation. Other common errors involve drug-drug interactions or failure to monitor serious side effects. Many of these errors are clinically relevant, and 5%–10% result in potentially serious or life-threatening harm.

One of the most effective means of enhancing medication safety is the use of electronic prescribing with templates, built-in warnings, and stop-gaps to ensure that clinically significant interactions and errors are detected at the time of prescription. A nonpunitive culture around reporting potential or actual errors should be espoused to allow for timely reporting and adjustment of medication safety practices. Close involvement of clinical and pharmacy staff in drug monitoring and use, as well as regular monitoring of the literature for published reports of adverse drug reactions, can affect the provision of care. This practice should be incorporated into your multidisciplinary team meetings to ensure review of medication safety as a regular practice in patient care.

Race and Ethnicity Gap

Racial and ethnic minorities, particularly African American persons, tend to have greater and more persistent mental illness and use inpatient psychiatric services at a higher rate with increased risk for poor aftercare and readmission. Despite illness severity being a significant risk factor for readmission and a marker of service need, overall illness severity is not correlated with follow-up in racial and ethnic minorities. This provides an opportunity to enhance follow-up and reduce readmission among racial and ethnic minorities through greater integration, collaboration, and coordination between medical and psychiatric services.

Community factors affect inpatient psychiatric care for racial and ethnic minorities, particularly the availability of and access to evidence-based treatment, as well as stigma against pursuing mental health care. This also is affected by religious and cultural factors and suggests a key role for local community and spiritual leaders in identifying patients' needs and values and facilitating care. Strategies that have resulted in improved inpatient and postdischarge care include discharge planning in conjunction with outpatient providers, implementation of outpatient programming while continuing to receive inpatient care, engaging family in care, use of care coordination, and increasing meaningful supports in the health system.

Consultation Psychiatry and Integrated Care

The opportunity for quality improvement is tremendous in collaborative and integrated care settings. Psychiatric disorders cause significant disability and constitute four of the top six diseases affecting quality-adjusted life years as documented by the World Health Organization (Goldman et al. 2015). Comorbid psychiatric and physical illness can significantly compound issues related to access to, use of, and quality of care. Mental illness is a significant factor in high use of inpatient services and is a strong contributor to 30-day readmission rates. Patients with mental and physical health comorbidity are more likely to be hospitalized than are patients with only mental or only physical illness (Chen et al. 2016). Among medically hospitalized patients, one-third of the patients at a given time have active mental health issues, mostly comorbid depression or anxiety. Medically hospitalized patients with any psychiatric or cognitive comorbidity use medical resources at a higher rate with longer hospital stays, more procedures, and increased cost (Koopmans et al. 2005; Levenson et al. 1990; Saravay et al. 1991). Integrated care models have been shown to reduce costs and improve quality of care, particularly in high-need populations. Despite the growing evidence establishing the value of integration, the incentives for linkages between mental and physical health systems are sparse, and research and effort exploring best practices in integration and outcome assessment have been limited.

The focused, disease-specific process measures that compose a large proportion of existing quality measures in psychiatric care do not fully capture the opportunities to assess quality in integrated care settings. Consultation-liaison (C-L) psychiatry has a tremendous opportunity to bridge gaps in care at the interface of physical and mental health. C-L services can improve outcomes for medically hospitalized patients who have psychiatric comorbidity with reductions in length of stay, cost, morbidity, and mortality. Despite this, C-L referral rates are lower than 5% in inpatient medical settings. Barriers to referral include lack of psychiatrist availability, limited consultation resources, constraints on consultant time, poor communication, inadequate recognition of mental health needs, and minimal familiarity with mental health services among consultee services.

Fundamental to increased C-L referral is the quality of your longitudinal, regular engagement with care teams. C-L services that are active and communicative and work closely with their consultees tend to have greater use of their services with improved communication and outcomes. These working relationships can be enhanced through direct care but also

TABLE 15–3. Factors related to improved consultee satisfaction with the consultation experience

---

Consultant shows understanding of the clinical situation and core question being asked.

Consultation occurs within 24 hours of consult placement.

Consultant provides practical and helpful management recommendations to consultee and to nurses.

Consultant quickly manages patient behavioral difficulties.

Consultant verbally communicates recommendations directly to the consultee in addition to writing notes in the chart.

Consultant provides diagnostic clarification, effective management, and disposition planning.

Consultant facilitates timely transfer to inpatient psychiatry or other appropriate mental health dispositions.

After initial consultation, consultant provides follow-up within appropriate time to address patient's behavioral difficulties.

---

through your provision of education; regular communication with the entire care team, including social workers, nurses, other staff, and trainees; and offering the regular message that the C-L service is "available and ready to assist." Mid-level providers, nurses, social workers, and residents or fellow trainees can be important groups to target for education and relationship building because these individuals spend more time at the bedside and are at the front lines in detecting mental illness. Once the relationships are established and nurtured through collaborative care, educational activities, quality improvement, and research, the quality of those relationships and the care delivered will encourage referrals.

C-L psychiatry involves two consumers of the care experience: the patient receiving the care and the consultee who made the referral. Failure to attend to both consumers can result in declining referral to the service. Therefore, consultee satisfaction is just as important as patient satisfaction (Table 15–3). Consultees are more impressed by your understanding of the issues at hand and the questions being asked; longitudinal follow-up and collaboration; and provision of helpful diagnostic, management, and referral recommendations than they are by the speed of the consultation.

It is critical that consultees be able to detect mental illness, with education and training being a key factor in C-L service. A positive association is found between self-perceived abilities to manage psychiatric issues and lower referral rates, which may be a result of reduced knowledge or awareness of mental illness or lower prioritization of mental illness. This emphasizes the important role of the "L" in "C-L," with liaison work and education of our colleagues in medicine critical to the value and viability of a C-L service.

Developing Consensus Regarding Core Quality Measures

With growing interest in quality assessment and improvement, there has been a proliferation of quality measures with varying utility and value. Given the heterogeneity and inconsistent application of these measures, hospitals, payers, and legislators have advocated for the use of "core" measures. These measures are select, high-yield performance measures with clearly defined parameters that are generalizable, meaningful to all invested parties, feasible, and sustainable. Little agreement exists on common core measures, and without consensus, the result has been variability in data collection, limited comparability between settings, slower innovation, and limited refinement of quality measurement and improvement efforts.

Development of a set of core measures reduces cost in measurement and reporting of quality measures, and comparators across settings spur improved care and increased innovation. However, the development of core measures assumes that there are potential metrics that meet a broad array of criteria, can be used for multiple purposes, and are agreeable to a highly diverse group of stakeholders. The characteristics of a given quality measure and the aspects of the mental health system being assessed need to be considered simultaneously. Inherent in development of core measures are the conflicts between optimization of measure utility and broadening generalizability. The value of a performance measure can be highly subjective and may be skewed by the stakeholder, so the evidence must support both the accuracy and the value of the performance measure.

Once measures have been identified, maximization of the use of those measures is fraught with the difficulties of specification. What input, process, or outcome is to be assessed? Over what time frame? What population? Are there any inclusion or exclusion criteria? What setting or settings? What data sources? Many cumbersome questions raise further points of contention. Even if these measures are well defined, they need mechanisms to abstract, input, and report data. Further processes need to ensure the accuracy of the data being collected. This can be challenging because of the structures, personnel, and resources within different settings.

Ultimately, cost and resource utilization are often the largest barriers to core measure selection and implementation, largely based on the feasibility and sustainability of that measure. Furthermore, although a measure may be well defined, broadly applied, and accurate, the measure still may not be implemented because of difficulty interpreting results, limited control over an aspect of care confounding outcomes, or a lack of tangible improvements in care.

Measures also require a consensus norm for performance to meet a given quality standard. Complete adoption of a performance measure may be an expectation for some aspects of care, such as lethality assessments, but often a percent adherence to a given measure is expected. Norms reflect the average result or outcome of a given care setting, whereas benchmarks are measures used to assess the best-performing care settings compared with other less-performing settings. The use of comparative data to interpret quality measures can have a significant effect on provider behavior and perception of performance, making it all the more important to choose measures carefully.

Yet few benchmarks and norms exist in mental health, and those that do exist often meet only the minimum standards needed to provide acceptable, evidence-based care. We must engage in this process more actively, more thoughtfully, and in a more sustained way. Above all, we must use the data we collect to improve our care through the innovation and follow-up assessment that constitute continuous quality improvement.

KEY POINTS

- In the age of managed care, there is a pressing need to improve transparency in care, reduce costs, support patient- and family-centered care models, and improve quality of care.

- The inpatient psychiatric care setting provides unique challenges but equally unique opportunities to address quality improvement issues.

- Although the mental health evidence base in quality improvement and assessment is small relative to other disciplines and settings, it is rapidly growing with clear tenets to the selection and use of quality measures.

- A careful approach to the use of quality measures that are feasible, sustainable, and meaningful can enhance reporting, inform patients in their care, and incentivize quality improvement for providers.

- As greater consensus is reached across health systems, standards of quality will become more commonplace. It is important for psychiatric hospitalists to take the lead in this process.

- The potential is great and with greater understanding of and engagement in quality improvement, the psychiatric hospitalist can be actively involved in shaping how quality is assessed and reported and the effect quality improvement may have on care delivery and outcomes.

References

Chen KY, Evans R, Larkins S: Why are hospital doctors not referring to consultation-liaison psychiatry? - a systemic review. BMC Psychiatry 16:390, 2016 27829386

Goldman ML, Spaeth-Rublee B, Pincus HA: Quality indicators for physical and behavioral health integration. JAMA 314:769–770, 2015 26043185

Koopmans GT, Donker MCH, Rutten FHH: Length of hospital stay and health service use of medical inpatients with comorbid noncognitive mental disorders: a review of the literature. Gen Hosp Psychiatry 27:44–56, 2005 15694218

Levenson JL, Hamer RM, Rossiter LF: Relation of psychopathology in general medical inpatients to use and cost of services. Am J Psychiatry 147:1498–1503, 1990 2121054

Saravay SM, Steinberg MD, Weinschel B, et al: Psychological comorbidity and length of stay in the general hospital. Am J Psychiatry 148:324–329, 1991 1992834

CHAPTER 16
Patient Safety

Katrina Bozada, M.D.
Laura Hirshbein, M.D., Ph.D.

According to the World Health
Organization, patient safety is "a framework of organized activities that creates cultures, processes, procedures, behaviours, technologies and environments in health care that consistently and sustainably lower risks, reduce the occurrence of avoidable harm, make error less likely and reduce its impact when it does occur" (World Health Organization 2021, p. 1). In the last few decades, American physicians and policy analysts have stressed the importance of safety in health care settings, especially hospitals. Organizations such as the Institute of Medicine have reported that errors in hospitals have led to patient injury and death, and a culture of safety is being promoted by individuals and organizations to try to reduce medical error. The assumption behind most initiatives in this area has been that although hospital staffs are composed of humans who can make mistakes, everyone shares the goal of improving the safety of the environment. These include concerns for the proper use of medications, avoidance of medication errors, and reconciliation of inpatient medications with discharge orders; treatment of medical conditions (both previous and new onset); and recognition, avoidance, and treatment of other iatrogenic issues.

For psychiatric patients, the phrase *patient safety* includes not only harm *to* a patient but also harm *by* a patient to himself or herself or others during the process of treatment. In this respect, the practice of psychiatric medicine differs from other medical disciplines and is held to additional standards. This is not to say that other medical specialties do not need to think about these safety concerns. Screening and safety assessments for suicide are required by regulatory bodies and are ideally performed during initial intakes in the emergency department and other outpatient settings. In addition, inpatient providers in other medical specialties need to remain vigilant for the development of these safety concerns during the treatment of their patients. The potential for dangerousness to self and others, however, is a constant issue in the treatment of patients on a psychiatric unit and one that helps frame a multitude of decisions from treatment options to length of stay and discharge planning.

Dangerousness to Self and Others

As resources have become more scarce and outpatient mental health treatment is harder to come by, the hospital has become a more important mediator in a broad spectrum of patient mental health issues. People who are experiencing a mental health crisis and cannot find any outpatient treatment might come to the emergency department because there seem to be few options available. Parents whose children made statements about suicide in school come to emergency departments to get evaluations. Patients who report worsening symptoms of their schizophrenia or bipolar disorder might come in because they are having side effects of medications. Severely ill patients might be brought in by police if they are acting out in the community. Patients who have made suicide attempts require emergency treatment and sometimes medical stabilization before their psychiatric issues can be addressed.

In addition to the volume and acuity that characterize hospital settings, economic issues are further shaping the intensity of the hospital environment. As hospitalizations are being managed more by outside entities (such as insurance companies or community mental health organizations), hospitalized patients are becoming more and more acutely ill. Because authorization criteria for hospitalization are increasingly limited to patients with acute risk for dangerousness to self or others, the number of high-risk patients admitted to inpatient psychiatric hospitals continues to increase. The economic pressures also push for quick resolution of safety issues and rapid stabilization and discharge from the hospital.

Given the high intensity of psychiatric settings—and of psychiatric patients in medical settings—it is critical to assess for safety of patients toward themselves and others. It is not enough to simply ask patients whether they are thinking about harming themselves or others (although this unfortunately seems to be the focus of many insurance reviewers). Instead, you need to be attentive to the environment, the frequent types of patient presentations, the immediate and longer-term warning signs (especially agitation), and the ways in which we can manage risk as much as possible.

Assessment of Dangerousness

Suicide Risk Assessment

Suicide risk assessment is a component of every hospital-based psychiatric evaluation and subsequent patient interaction. Many hospital systems use the Columbia-Suicide Severity Rating Scale or other formal instruments to assist staff in screening for patients who have had thoughts of suicide. As a psychiatrist, components of your suicide risk assessment begin with an introduction to the topic and straightforward questions about thoughts of suicide ranging from passive ideas of not waking from sleep or falling prey to an accident to thoughts of specific ways of ending one's life, making plans to act, and degree of intent to act. Patients who are disturbed by these thoughts and actively seeking treatment will welcome the opportunity to share them and engage in treatment to address them. Other patients who are seeking to avoid treatment, either to enable them to act on their suicidal thoughts or to leave the hospital for other reasons, such as to continue substance use, will deny these thoughts and plans. In these cases, it is essential that you seek as much information about the patient's recent condition, behavior, and entry into the hospital as possible. It is permissible to do so even without the patient's consent. Only after taking these steps is it reasonable to conclude that a patient poses low risk for self-harm. Patients who have spoken to others about or previously acted on undisclosed suicidal thoughts may become more amenable to discussion after being confronted with the observations of family and friends, police reports, or medical test results. For those who continue to deny their intent despite obvious evidence of suicidality, involuntary admission may be the only option. (For more on this topic, see Chapter 14, "Legal and Ethical Issues.")

Assessment of Assault Risk

Assessment of assault risk follows much the same pattern as suicide risk assessment, with the addition of observations of the patient's thought process, speech, and behavior. Although some assaultive behavior is contemplated and planned in much the same way that suicidal behavior often is, in hospital settings it is usually impulsive and driven by agitation, anger, cognitive disorganization, and impulsivity. Evidence of these may be apparent in aggressive acts before or during arrival at the hospital, loud or threatening comments, muscle tension, or obvious anger. Long-term history is especially important in these cases because previous assaultive behavior is a reliable predictor of future risk.

Dangerousness in the Emergency Department

Emergency departments are perhaps the most dangerous places among all health care settings. Patients arrive to the emergency department through a variety of means, including walk-ins, referrals from outside providers, ambulance, or even police, and the diverse symptoms require hospital staff to adapt quickly to patients who are often unfamiliar to them with unpredictable behaviors. In addition, the department must be ready for the possibility of more than one patient to be acutely dangerous at any point in time and have procedures in place for how to handle such active milieus. In the emergency setting, patient conditions are acute, and they can present with both medical and psychiatric symptoms. Medical concerns should be worked up and treated accordingly, and when appropriate, medical admission with psychiatric consultation should be considered.

Environmental factors are another consideration in this setting. Emergency departments are busy places that are often noisy and crowded. This can add further distress to already anxious and depressed individuals who are considering harming themselves or feed into the paranoia of psychotic patients who may react to protect themselves from perceived harm. Some hospitals may have separate, dedicated psychiatric emergency services to house individuals undergoing psychiatric evaluations, but most do not. In these cases, care should be taken to use quieter areas of the emergency department, to remove unnecessary equipment from these rooms, and to provide patient sitters or attendants.

Patient aggression toward caregivers is one of the most challenging aspects of emergency care. It is extremely helpful when approaching agitated patients to employ a provider team that uses similar behavioral safety techniques and effectively communicates not only with one another but with the patient. Emergency staff aim to provide ideal care and to intervene as necessary to prevent adverse outcomes such as suicide, but the realities of busy clinical practices can interfere with aspirations.

Dangerousness in Transitions of Care

Vignette

Mr. R, a 36-year-old man, has a history of paranoid schizophrenia. He had been off his medications for more than a year before he was brought to the emergency department by his mother who was worried because he seemed increasingly paranoid and disorganized. Mr. R was superficially cooperative with the emergency evaluation process, but he continued to insist that he did not need to be in the hospital. He had a prolonged wait time in the emergency department because of a lack of psychiatric hospital beds. Nursing staff members felt bad about how long he was cooped up in a secure area. At his request, they took him outside for some fresh air in a wheelchair. As soon as they got outside, the patient jumped out of the wheelchair and ran off. Staff members were unable to catch him, and it was not clear how they would have intervened had they done so.

Once a decision about disposition of a patient has been made, there is further risk that the patient will act out intentionally or unintentionally as a result of unhappiness with the plan. Some patients concur with whatever the plan is from the emergency department—admission or discharge. Others are less agreeable. A psychotic patient might be unhappy about being admitted to a hospital and be argumentative and agitated. A patient with an opiate use disorder might be angry that he is not getting a prescription for opiates in the emergency department. A patient might be so psychotic and disorganized that she is striking out at everyone because she thinks someone is trying to poison her.

The biggest risks in these situations are that the patient might strike out at a provider, run away, or be superficially cooperative but then act out more aggressively at the next level of care. It is optimal to have a mobile hospital security team that can work with clinic staff to allow them to feel safe as they calmly and clearly communicate with patients what can (or cannot) happen next. If a security team is not available or a more flexible system of response to agitated patients is needed, the staff should be trained in some kind of nonviolent intervention (with or without training in physical management) so that everyone is in agreement about how things should work in the case of an aggressive patient. It is essential that in a crisis, the team has a shared and clear understanding of who is responsible for what and who is in charge.

Without a secured space, there is a risk of elopement. Sometimes patients will appear cooperative but are carefully searching for opportunities to get away. This risk can be managed with either sufficient staff to watch at-risk patients or a monitoring system that will set off alarms if a patient leaves an area. However a hospital system manages a patient who is unhappy or acting out, it is essential to make sure that all of the staff understand what is happening. This means that the events within the emergency department need to be clearly conveyed to an accepting inpatient unit.

Dangerousness in Medical-Surgical Units

Screening for Suicide Risk

Screening for suicide risk should be done on a routine basis either with all admitted patients or with those who were admitted with injuries that could have been self-inflicted. Patients who score positive on screening measures or who acknowledge self-injurious behaviors should be seen by a psychiatrist. Not all patients who have had thoughts of suicide or injured themselves require psychiatric hospitalization, and the psychiatric consultation service can more expertly assess what level of care is necessary for the patient and also help the medical or surgical teams understand the next steps.

Aggressive Behavior Due to Medical Causes

Aggressive behavior due to medical causes is often interpreted as a psychiatric problem for which a hospital seeks the solution via admission to a psychiatric unit. Much of the time this is not appropriate, however. Patients receiving postoperative care who are delirious, hallucinating, and striking out are not at all appropriate for an inpatient psychiatric unit. A consultation service can help the medical teams understand the value of verbal redirection and a patient sitter to help keep the patient oriented. A consultation psychiatrist can also educate medical and surgical teams about the appropriate timing and dosage of antipsychotic medications that can be used for agitation.

Safety of the Environment

Safety of the environment on a medical or surgical unit cannot be assumed for a suicidal or self-harming patient. Many potential environmental hazards are found, including tubing, intravenous needles, silverware from meal trays, curtains, and alcohol-based hand sanitizer. The safest way to monitor patients who are at significant risk for self-harm or suicide but who cannot (yet) be transitioned to an inpatient psychiatric unit is to have a patient attendant or sitter. The patient attendants need to be trained to observe patients, to recognize common warning signs for self-harm behaviors, and to know what steps to take to intervene.

Dangerousness in Inpatient Psychiatric Units

Vignette

Ms. J, a 33-year-old woman with a long history of mood instability, substance abuse, and self-harm behaviors, was admitted through the emergency department at the recommendation of her outpatient psychiatrist. The psychiatrist was worried about the patient's pattern of impulsivity and her reports of worsening distress, increased self-harm, and thoughts of overdose. Ms. J was admitted voluntarily and participated in the adult psychiatry inpatient unit admission protocol, including a property search and a comprehensive skin check. On the second day of her hospitalization, Ms. J handed her nurse a note informing him that she had overdosed on aripip-razole (not a medication she was being given in the hospital). On the recommendation of Poison Control, Ms. J was transferred to a medical floor and monitored on telemetry for a day with no serious medical issues. A urine screen was negative for aripiprazole, but the patient produced pills that she had hidden in her room. On readmission to the psychiatry unit, Ms. J stated that she had smuggled in the pills (hidden in the lining of her underwear). She was vague on the question of whether she brought the pills with an intention of dying but did say that she wanted to have medication available in case she felt anxious because she was convinced that staff at the hospital would not take her reports of anxiety seriously or adequately respond to her. Ms. J was psychiatrically stabilized after several more days and was discharged to her outpatient provider.

Environmental Security

Environmental security is the first step in making sure that patients are safe on an inpatient unit. The unit as a whole should already be set up with environmental factors taken into consideration to reduce risk for suicide on the unit (e.g., door alarms, furniture and wall structures with reduced ligature points) as well as procedures in place to continue actively looking for and correcting these risks. The number one method of completed suicide on an inpatient unit is asphyxiation via strangulation, hanging, or suffocation. Special precautions need to be in place to guard against each of these possibilities. These include use of cordless telephones and other electronic devices, removal of belts and shoelaces, and frequent direct observation of the patient.

Patient Acuity

Patient acuity is not based on what a patient says he or she is going to do. The most vulnerable time for suicide is shortly after admission, especially in times of heightened patient agitation. Suicide remains one of the top 10 leading causes of death in the United States, a reported 48–65 of which occur in the inpatient setting annually (Williams et al. 2018). Suicide is one of the top sentinel events reviewed by The Joint Commission, on par with falls and wrong-site surgery. Therefore, the suicide risk assessment needs to continue throughout the patient's stay, including multiple times a day by various providers.

On an inpatient unit, the patient's treatment team often consists of physicians, social workers, nurses, and activity or group therapists. It is important that the treatment team communicates with one another via treatment team meetings, in notes, and in person to express changes in the patient's risk status and treatment planning. Although patients are often seen as being in a protected environment during their admission, they are still subject to acute psychosocial stressors from the outside world. During the course of a patient's stay, bad news is often given to a patient by family (e.g., divorce, separation), relationships (e.g., breakups), roommates (e.g., housing loss), work supervisors (e.g., job loss, forced leave), and even outside psychiatric providers (e.g., termination of care, which forces these discussions and subsequent referrals on the inpatient treatment team). It is often out of the treatment team's control when other people share this information with patients, which often happens during telephone calls or visiting hours when most of the treatment team is not present. Sometimes, this news is shared directly with the inpatient treatment team who then has to navigate decisions on how and when to share certain news with patients. A variety of factors inform these decisions and often are individualized to patients based on history of distress tolerance, coping abilities, and other known risks. One thing to keep in mind is the timing of such news by the treatment team; it would not be a good idea to pass on news at the end of the day when most providers are leaving. It is important that the unit has guidelines in place for initiating and responding to changes in a patient at acute risk for harm to self, including for suicide and self-injurious behavior no matter the time of day or shift.

Inappropriate Sexual Interactions

Inappropriate sexual interactions between patients can represent safety issues. Consensual sexual behaviors occur on inpatient units despite a unit's rules restricting these types of behaviors and may even occur undetected by staff. Factors that may contribute to consensual relationships on inpatient psychiatric units include the vulnerability of patients during a time of heightened emotions and the patient's own psychiatric symptoms, which may include hypersexuality and impulsive behaviors (e.g., manic or borderline personality disorder patients). However, even consensual relationships may have adverse consequences, including transmission of sexually transmitted diseases and pregnancy. In addition, sexual behavior, both consensual and nonconsensual, may cause trauma and interfere with treatment. Nonconsensual sexual behaviors include public exposure of genitalia or masturbation, inappropriate touching, and sexual assault. Both patients and staff are susceptible to these types of interactions.

Discharge Planning

The risk for suicide is high in the days and weeks following discharge from an inpatient unit. Given these risks, during an inpatient admission, the focus is often on helping suicidal patients with treatment modalities such as therapy and medications as well as safety planning for discharge to help mitigate this risk.

In preparing for discharge, there are many potential pitfalls as teams work with human patients (e.g., patients are unpredictable and not always fully forthcoming with their plans). In busy hospital settings, sometimes patients put pressure on teams for discharge that in hindsight was rushed or unsafe. Teams may fail to communicate effectively with outpatient providers and families about the level of risk. Sometimes patients do not make it to their next level of care.

Medication Safety and Iatrogenic Complications

Vignette

Mr. K, a 63-year-old man with a long history of bipolar disorder, was admitted to the psychiatric unit because of manic symptoms. He had not been sleeping in days and was impressively grandiose. He was making plans to donate a great deal of money to different staff members in the hospital and spoke about celebrities he called "dear friends" (even though he had never met them). Mr. K was given escalating doses of a second-generation antipsychotic with no visible effect after several days. A mood stabilizer was added, along with frequent doses of a benzodiazepine. Despite all of this medication, the patient appeared to get more disorganized and slept even less. He began to slur his words and had a hard time recognizing staff. He significantly improved after the antipsychotic was discontinued and the benzodiazepine doses were reduced.

One of the main ways in which we manage acute agitation in the hospital is through the use of medications. In addition, we rapidly titrate medications such as mood stabilizers or antipsychotics for highly symptomatic patients. Complicated alcohol withdrawal is treated with generous use of benzodiazepines, and we continue medications for issues such as high blood pressure, diabetes, and chronic pain. In this subsection, we focus on ways that we can address systems and environmental issues to try to minimize medication problems and other hospital-acquired issues.

Nonpharmacological Methods of Addressing Inpatient Issues

Nonpharmacological methods of addressing inpatient issues tend to be overlooked in managing acute problems. For better or for worse, both physicians and nurses have high regard for medications and their effects, and some hospital clinicians can get into a pattern of prescribing rather than talking to patients. But it is better for patients (and ultimately better for the staff) to start with other kinds of interventions. Patients should be asked when they are admitted what kinds of things help them calm down when they are upset. If that is not possible, the information about nonmedication interventions should be obtained from chart review or conversation with families (if permitted with privacy laws in the state). Hospital teams might use distractions such as drawing or music to help patients de-escalate without medications. Avoidance of medications, although not free of risk, is the first line of defense against the adverse effects of psychotropics.

Common Iatrogenic Treatment Issues

Common iatrogenic treatment issues include delirium from excessive use of medication combinations and high doses of medications. Sedating medications, such as benzodiazepines, anticholinergics, and antipsychotics, are especially prone to induce delirium. Patients with alcohol withdrawal are at risk for delirium because of both the withdrawal and the benzodiazepines given. Patients undergoing electroconvulsive therapy may experience delirium in addition to disorientation and memory loss.

Other iatrogenic symptoms that occur most frequently in hospital settings are acute dystonic reactions from antipsychotics because of the prevalence of medication initiation, rapid dose titration, and high total doses. Neuroleptic malignant syndrome is likewise most prevalent with initiation or rapid escalation of antipsychotic doses. Serotonergic symptoms may occur in patients given vigorous doses of serotonergic antidepressants. Serious drug interactions are not common with psychiatric medications but may occur when several serotonergic medications are given or when drugs interfere with each other's metabolism.

Fall Risk

Fall risk can be heightened, especially in older patients, on inpatient services in a new environment with unfamiliar floor surfaces, room layouts, bed design, and bathroom structure. Many units require patients to relinquish shoes with laces (to avoid strangulation risk), so patients are wearing either slip-on shoes or socks. In addition, there is a significant risk of psychiatric medications having side effects that can result in falls. Medications may cause sedation, anticholinergic effects, dizziness, hypotension, or reduced alertness, all things that can make falls more likely. Patient bathrooms are places in which falls can be more likely because of slippery floors and transitions in and out of the shower. It is best if the entire team works together to minimize fall risk by providing signs for the patients to remind them to get up slowly, an environmental survey to reduce mobility hazards, and regular review of medications to reduce the risk for dizziness or disorientation.

Hospital-Acquired Infections

Hospital-acquired infections are less common on an inpatient psychiatric unit because antibiotics are used less frequently than elsewhere in the hospital, but psychiatric units need to participate in general infection prevention precautions, including contact or isolation precautions as needed. The most straightforward—but still challenging—intervention psychiatric hospital staff members can do is to wash or sanitize hands before and after patient contacts. This can feel odd and uncomfortable for experienced mental health professionals. Many of us in the past made a practice of just talking to patients and washing hands only before doing a physical examination. Those of us who routinely treat obsessive-compulsive disorder may consciously avoid framing patient encounters by obvious hand sanitizing before a conversation. But this is one area in which the hospital's larger goal of patient safety has to override older psychodynamic issues. Hospitals can be places in which germs flourish. With apologies to our patients with obsessive-compulsive disorder tendencies, it is good practice (and a regulatory requirement) to wash hands before and after each patient encounter.

Less Common (but Still Worrisome) Risks

Less common (but still worrisome) risks include the potential for deep venous thrombosis and pulmonary embolism in hospitalized patients. This risk is aggressively addressed on medical-surgical floors, but no reliable data indicate how to address this risk in psychiatric inpatients. For medical and surgical patients, the first level of prevention for a thrombosis is to use sequential compression devices, which are inflatable bladders that wrap around the legs to compress them and reduce the chance of blood clots. In a psychiatric setting, however, these are impractical, may interfere with treatment, and use tubing that raises the risk for self-harm behaviors. Many patients are active on an inpatient unit (much more so than on medical floors), substantially reducing the risk, but others may spend significant time immobile as a result of depression, catatonia, or electroconvulsive therapy recovery. In these cases, anticoagulation may be appropriate.

KEY POINTS

- One of the primary responsibilities of the psychiatric hospitalist is patient safety, requiring attention both to individual patients and to systems of care.

- The major safety issue for psychiatric patients is dangerousness to self and others.

- Assessment of suicidality and assault risk is a primary responsibility of the hospital-based psychiatrist and must be conducted systematically, thoroughly, and regularly.

- Agitation is an additional key component of risk of harm to self and others.

- Hospital teams in the emergency department, transitions of care, medical-surgical units, and inpatient psychiatric units need to have clear protocols to manage acute agitation to minimize the risk to patients and staff.

References

Williams SC, Schmaltz SP, Castro GM, Baker DW: Incidence and method of suicide in hospitals in the United States. Jt Comm J Qual Patient Saf 44(11):643–650, 2018 30190221

World Health Organization: Patient safety. 2021. Available at: www.who.int/health-topics/patient-safety#tab=tab_1. Accessed June 15, 2021.

CHAPTER 17
Adverse Events

Michael D. Jibson, M.D., Ph.D.

Adverse events are unfavorable outcomes attributable to a fault in medical care. The underlying assumptions that distinguish an adverse event from other negative outcomes are that 1) the outcome would have been preventable with appropriate care and 2) a failure to provide that care resulted in harm to the patient. Adverse events are widespread and significantly contribute to morbidity and mortality in all fields of medicine, including mental health. Suicides, attempted suicides, assaults, medication side effects, injuries with restraints, unexpected deaths, falls, and elopements are among the incidents most commonly categorized as adverse events during psychiatric care.

Preventable or unexpected incidents with the most serious outcomes, such as a patient's death, permanent injury, or extreme temporary harm, are defined by The Joint Commission as "sentinel events." Examples of sentinel events in hospitals include amputation of the wrong limb, discharge of a newborn to the wrong family, or transfusion of incompatible blood. Two such sentinel events belong specifically to psychiatry: suicide within 72 hours of discharge from a hospital or emergency department and serious self-inflicted injury on a hospital service.

Other adverse events are usually categorized by the seriousness of their outcome. A spectrum of severity among suicide attempts, self-injury, and other harm extends from superficial scratches to near-lethal results. Both the emotional and the administrative response to these occurrences will be proportional to the injury, or potential for injury, that resulted. As a hospital-based psychiatrist, you are likely to encounter these events both as a clinician and as an expert called on to orchestrate an appropriate response. In this chapter, I review those responses rather than the patient safety issues these events may highlight, which were discussed in Chapter 16, "Patient Safety."

Risk Management

The hospital's response to an adverse event falls under the rubric of risk management, which includes the investigation, review, and corrective action required to address the individual event and recommendations for changes that will prevent its recurrence. Although much of this activity is directed toward reduction of legal liability, it also includes preventive actions to avoid medical errors and quality improvement activities to optimize patient care (see Chapter 15, "Quality Assessment and Improvement"). Most hospitals have an office devoted to risk management, regardless of whether they use that name. Alternatively, if you work within a hospital but not for the hospital, as in some private practice settings, your malpractice insurer will have a risk management program ready to assist you. You will do well to become familiar with this group and their functions before an untoward event occurs and to engage their services as soon as possible afterward.

Communication

The first step to address a major adverse event is to open lines of communication within the hospital among the various clinicians involved, with hospital administration, and with the patient and family. Communication with hospital administration usually will occur via the Risk Management Office, which should be notified as quickly as possible. They will not only advise you on the appropriate steps to take but also facilitate communication and ensure that appropriate medical, administrative, and legal resources are available.

Simultaneously, you should notify your clinical director to inform him or her of the event and to seek specific direction that he or she may have. Contact among clinicians may be restricted to the members of your treatment team or may cross services and specialties. Notification of involved clinicians is essential but often haphazard in a large and complex health care system. A quick review of medical notes will yield an initial list of individuals to contact with news of the event. In the case of a death, particularly a death by suicide, it may be appropriate to reach out to clinicians formerly involved as well, rather than leave them unaware or to learn through other means.

For trainees, in addition to the clinical supervisor, the director of the medical student clerkship or residency program should be apprised. Students and residents generally are not familiar with how adverse events are handled and invariably feel intense vulnerability in these situations. Early contact with their program leadership will reassure them that supervisors have final responsibility for patient care and will be there to support them.

Surviving patients and families should be contacted promptly, informed as specifically as possible about what has happened, and invited to meet personally. Even a brief warning of impending bad news may help the family cope with the loss of a loved one. If emergency procedures, such as an attempt to resuscitate a patient, are in progress, take the opportunity to contact the family while the procedure is under way. Telling them that their loved one has developed a serious medical problem that the hospital's emergency response team is trying to address is a better option than either giving or withholding news of a death in an initial telephone contact. Meet personally with the family, hear their concerns, and give accurate and detailed information without speculation or implication of blame. Give them an opportunity to respond, assess their emotional state, and offer whatever support services are available. Subsequent communication with the family may be appropriate or may be better handled by either social work or risk management staff, depending on their needs (not your level of comfort).

Advice and Protection

Happily, adverse events are rare in the life of the individual clinician, even in a setting as acute as most hospital services. Consequently, most psychiatrists have little experience with the policies and procedures that guide the clinician and govern the hospital's response. News of an unfavorable outcome is invariably distressing and often an unexpected shock, leaving even senior practitioners stunned and off-balance. Risk management staff can help you navigate during the difficult period that follows such an event.

Special legal protections apply to communications and actions taken under the official auspices of quality assurance. Your involvement of the designated Risk Management Office allows those protections to apply to many of the critical tasks that will follow, including the communications described in the previous subsection. Both written and verbal conversations, when involving risk management or other designated quality assurance personnel, may be protected from the legal process of discovery, allowing for more candid discussion of the event than would be possible otherwise. Although this protection is not absolute and varies somewhat from state to state, it provides you with a significant measure of assurance that speculative comments, premature conclusions, or expressions of emotional distress will not outweigh more measured and thoughtful assessments of the event.

Legal Action

Fears of malpractice allegations play prominently in the consciousness of any clinician who has experienced a significant adverse event. Unfortunately, in today's litigious society, the threat of civil action is real and adds an additional locus of distress. The risk that is managed by the Risk Management Office is mostly legal, and your early contact with that office will assist you not only in communicating with other professionals and navigating hospital procedures but also by bearing the brunt of legal concerns and addressing these with the injured patient or deceased patient's family.

As legal issues play out, the risk management staff will be responsible for addressing and resolving them, including by involvement of attorneys or other legal advisers as may be appropriate. They will attempt to remedy the situation without a formal lawsuit if possible and will handle a lawsuit that does occur. They will make their own determination as to whether a financial settlement is required and will oversee any negotiations that may be involved. Should a court case ensue, they will take the lead both in responding to legal requirements and in preparing you for any role you may have to play, such as giving a deposition or court testimony. Although there may be situations in which the hospital's interests diverge from those of the individual physician, they are more often aligned, and your trust of and cooperation with risk managers will serve you well.

Event Review

Every adverse event should undergo some type of review to clarify the facts of the incident, the persons and services involved, issues that may need to be addressed, and steps that may be appropriate in response. The nature of that review will vary depending on the severity of the event, the services involved, and what type and level of intervention may be required to address it.

Level of Review

At a minimum, every reported event is reviewed by at least one physician assigned by the hospital to handle this task. Most often, this will be either the service director or the chair of a committee with this responsibility. The purpose of this initial review is to determine the severity of the incident and whether further investigation is appropriate. Cases with significant harm or risk of harm or that suggest potential opportunities to improve systems of care are most appropriate for formal review. Per Joint Commission standards, cases judged to be sentinel events must be reviewed in detail.

 Reviews may be conducted at the level of the clinical service, the department, or the medical center. Relatively minor incidents are generally handled by the service on which they occur. These cases give the clinicians on-site an opportunity to revisit service policies and procedures, update training of staff, examine physical facilities, and consider changes to treatment procedures. Local reviews may be as simple as informal discussions among staff or may involve more formal procedures of information gathering, committee discussion, creation of a written action plan, and later follow-up on whether recommended changes were implemented.

 Cases of moderate severity are more often handled at the departmental level, often by a standing committee with ongoing responsibility for conducting these reviews. Members of a departmental committee have the advantages of expertise in the clinical area involved and the perspective that comes with experience in these investigations. Their familiarity to the clinicians involved may make the process less threatening, and their understanding of the clinical issues at play gives them unique insight into these cases.

 Sentinel events are often reviewed at the institutional level, as a reflection of both their seriousness and the need for a more objective review of clinical policies and procedures. A group representing the various interprofessional disciplines involved in psychiatric care, including physicians, nursing staff, and social workers, may be involved. These are usually individuals with extensive experience and often formal training in the dissection of these cases, who are skilled at understanding not only what happened but also why things went wrong. The downside of an institutional review is that most of those involved work outside psychiatry and may not have an accurate sense of the work you do or the standard practices in the field. The positive side is that they may have access to resources outside the department that could not be used otherwise.

Vignette

Dr. A shared her residents' concerns about patient and staff safety in the emergency department, but her requests for additional security staff were repeatedly met with reassurances that security were not far away and would respond promptly if called. During an overnight shift, Dr. B, a postgraduate year–2 resident, was called to assess a man with a history of criminal activity who had come in complaining of suicidal ideation. A social worker had seen the patient and initiated the legal process for involuntary admission if necessary, a common precaution in this setting. The patient had been calm and cooperative throughout the visit, the service was backed up with cases, and Dr. B was not optimistic about the time it would take to arrange a security standby to conduct the interview. Without warning, the patient leaped up, grabbed Dr. B around the neck, and began making threats to everyone nearby. A single security officer responded within the designated 5-minute response time and called for additional officers; within 7 minutes, others arrived. Seeing the officers, the patient immediately let go of Dr. B and allowed himself to be restrained.

When interviewed by a hospital committee unfamiliar with psychiatric emergencies, Drs. B and A had to spend much of their time educating the reviewers about the nature of psychiatric disorders, unpredictability of certain behaviors, frequency of involuntary hospitalization, and difference between agitated and antisocial violence. The day after the reviewers' report was submitted to the director of the hospital, Dr. A was invited to a meeting with the director and the chief of security and was told to "bring a wish list" of security measures, all of which were promptly implemented.

Information Gathering

If a formal review is to be conducted at the departmental or institutional level, an individual or small group will be assigned to gather and organize pertinent information. At a minimum, this will involve a review of medical records and interviews with the front-line clinicians involved in the case. In more complex cases, additional sources of information may be sought, including information from family members, clinic supervisors, previous care providers, or law enforcement personnel. Police reports, autopsy findings, and written communications (including suicide notes) may be obtained. The goal of this process is to gather enough information to reconstruct the events that occurred, the factors that led to those events, and the thinking that went into each decision that was made and action that was taken.

For clinicians who are already traumatized by the news of an adverse event, this process may feel threatening and intimidating. Most psychiatrists report repeated second-guessing of their clinical judgment and decision-making after such an event, and many already harbor a false certainty of error, with intense feelings of guilt regarding their failure to respond appropriately to some subtle hint of impending danger in their last interaction with the patient.

The interviewer, by contrast, is mostly trying to understand, not judge, the decisions and their outcomes. This needs to be made clear to the clinician and the interview conducted accordingly. The atmosphere should be supportive and the questions phrased in positive or neutral terms. Frequent reference to the medical record may stimulate recall of pertinent events, help both the clinician and the reviewer maintain an accurate timeline, and allow the clinician to clarify and contextualize the information recorded.

Event Report and Review

Information from all sources then must be compiled into a single narrative that incorporates each perspective gathered. The report should be framed objectively and without assumptions of wrongdoing. Discrepancies may be highlighted but should be taken as evidence of variant perceptions rather than of error or deception. The goal of the report is to create as complete and accurate a picture of the case as possible, incorporating the patient's longitudinal history, pertinent recent events in the patient's life, a summary of care provided, details of recent visits, and the clinician's assessment of the patient's recent condition and risk.

The report is intended to be a statement of facts, among which are the events and documents of the case, along with the perceptions, beliefs, opinions, plans, and expectations of the clinician as the case was conducted. These need to be separated from the clinician's subsequent reflections and judgments, which should be addressed in a separate process.

In most instances, a committee is responsible for the process from this point forward. The committee will review the facts of the case and form an opinion on what happened, what factors played a role in the events, and what vulnerabilities in the care system it may highlight. Although it is hoped that any errors or deficits in care that occurred will come to light, the purpose of the review is not to affix blame but to learn from the event and to identify areas in which the system of care can be improved.

Root Cause Analysis

Root cause analysis is a procedure whereby as many factors as possible that contributed to a bad outcome are identified, and then those that would have prevented the outcome if corrected are separated from those that were merely contributory. One approach to root cause analysis is to ask a series of "why" questions until a cause is reached that lends itself to intervention that will be broadly effective rather than helpful only in the current case. The strength of a root cause analysis is that it identifies at least one action item that can be addressed in response to an adverse event. Its weakness is that most events are multifactorial and involve a convergence of factors, making the identification of one as the root cause somewhat arbitrary. More concerning is its underlying assumption that all bad outcomes can be prevented by appropriately designed and implemented systems of care, a dubious proposition at best.

Medical Errors

Medical errors are the exception in psychiatric adverse events, but they do occur, most often related to omissions in care or documentation. Even when such an omission is uncovered, the appropriate response may well be a change in the care system to make similar oversights less likely. For example, a clinician conducting a suicide risk assessment may neglect to ask about firearms in the home, leading the review committee to recommend changes to the medical record system to include a template or reminder of the importance of doing so. Alternatively, the committee may recommend staff training in suicide assessment or may provide feedback on clinicians' risk assessments through chart reviews.

Individual Performance Reviews

Individual performance reviews also may be recommended in particularly serious cases of medical error. A performance review generally will examine a broad sample of the clinician's chart notes to evaluate the caliber and style of the clinical assessments, patterns of treatment, quality of documentation, and treatment outcomes. Results of such a review may highlight specific areas of deficiency or, conversely, may indicate that the bad outcome occurred despite a consistent pattern of high-quality care.

Action Plans

Careful review of an adverse event may seem largely pointless in the absence of a specific set of changes that will be put in place to avoid similar future outcomes. In fact, the opposite is often the case, and the primary benefit of the review may well be to address the distress of the clinicians involved. Here, as at other points in the review and discussion process, it is important to have a realistic view of psychiatric adverse events, to recognize the fundamental impossibility of predicting human behavior, and to understand the limits of mental health interventions.

With that in mind, it is also important to recognize flaws in how systems work, potential areas for additional training, deficits in quality of care, and other areas where performance could be improved. No system is without such issues. An effective action plan identifies areas that would benefit from change without recommending onerous policies or procedures that would not genuinely improve care or prevent future untoward events.

The ideal action plan is realistic, focused, and efficient, with a measurable outcome that can be readily monitored. For example, firearms in the home are a known risk factor for completed suicide. The standard of care in most communities is to ascertain whether the patient has access to such weapons and to recommend to the patient and family as part of a comprehensive safety plan that they be removed. If a case review has determined that this is not routinely occurring in clinic visits, an action plan that provides training to clinicians, establishes an expectation that this question will be part of every suicide risk assessment and its documentation, and uses the electronic medical record to monitor compliance would be both reasonable to implement and reasonably likely to enhance patient safety.

Vignette

Dr. F, a postgraduate year–2 resident new to the child psychiatric inpatient unit, was anxious about the unfamiliar patient population and clinical setting but excited about this new experience. He soon found himself surrounded by challenging clinical issues and a workload that left little time for reflection or detailed supervision. Faced with an urgent need to get an uncooperative 10-year-old to a required unit activity, he grabbed him by the arm and dragged him a few feet down the hall, where the sullen, but unharmed patient grudgingly participated in his therapy group. Unbeknownst to Dr. F, the encounter was video recorded on the monitor over the front door of the unit and soon came to the attention of security officers reviewing the recording, the unit director, the Patient Rights Office, and the patient's family. An adverse event review followed with an initial finding of wrongdoing by Dr. F. The review committee continued, however, with a root cause analysis, noting that Dr. F had acted improperly because of his unfamiliarity with hospital policies and unit priorities, he was unfamiliar with these policies because he had not been oriented at the beginning of the rotation, and he had not been oriented because of a long-standing pattern of inadequate trainee supervision on that service. Dr. F was required to go through additional patient rights training, but the committee also recommended that all residents have the training. More importantly, they recommended that higher standards of oversight be maintained on resident rotations, a measure welcomed by trainees and faculty alike.

Clinician Support

Among adverse events, suicide may be unique in its effect on clinicians. Other adverse events (such as a nonlethal injury) tend to be less stigmatized and consequential and arouse proportionally less intense feelings. Although it is highly debatable that all suicides are preventable, they are treated as such not only by Joint Commission policy but also by mental health providers whose response to a patient death tends overwhelmingly to include feelings of extreme guilt, failure, and loss of confidence. Typical responses include the certainty that there must have been clues, however subtle, to the coming tragedy; that some different word or action during the last contact with the patient would have led to a more favorable outcome; or that some real or imagined fault of the clinician will result in catastrophic professional consequences if exposed. These responses are common, normal, and intensely painful. It is essential that they be addressed through a variety of interventions.

Debriefing

Once the required notifications of the event have been made, attention to the well-being of the clinicians and staff members involved in the care of the patient becomes a high priority. One good strategy to address this need is to schedule a formal debriefing session as soon as possible after the event, open to anyone who felt connected to the case. Within the hospital setting, this tends to be many people, some of whom were not directly engaged in clinical tasks yet had some degree of responsibility for the patient's welfare. It is not unusual after an inpatient event not only for members of the primary physician team but also for nurses from multiple shifts, social workers, patient care workers, unit clerks, housekeeping staff, and unit administrators to want to be part of the discussion. One essential participant, who may choose to serve as facilitator, is a representative of the Risk Management Office, ensuring the status of the gathering as a quality assurance activity with the legal protection that carries.

The debrief may begin with the primary physician giving his or her perspective on what happened, followed by others who were directly involved sharing their own views of the event. This should allow a fairly complete picture of the event and serves to quell rumors and misinformation that may have circulated. It helps to clarify and consolidate memories and begins to establish a global narrative that will shape how the event is viewed over time.

The next equally important step is to allow those present to share their feelings about the case, such as the sadness, guilt, anger, compassion, or fears that were brought up by the event. Most often, this will be a chance for those with the most direct responsibility for the patient to expose their vulnerability and uncertainty and for those who work with them to offer support and consolation in much the same way that a high-functioning family behaves after the loss of a loved one. Less benign feelings also may be expressed, such as anger and blame directed at one another. This painful process also may be helpful to allow those feelings to be recognized and acknowledged. One session may be sufficient to address these issues, or additional gatherings may be scheduled to allow other staff to attend or to permit further processing of information and feelings.

Support Services

One advantage of work in a medical center is the possibility of an established physician support service for situations such as this. Significant attention has been directed to physician well-being, and one aspect of that is assistance following the loss of a patient to an event such as suicide. Services may include individual grief counseling or supportive therapy, general grief groups, or more focused support groups for clinicians following a patient suicide. Individual treatment may provide a safe framework for discussion of the clinician's feelings of guilt, loss, sadness, and inadequacy. Specialized groups may address the same issues while providing critical support from peers to normalize the experience and bolster confidence.

To be effective, these services must be readily available and ongoing. They must also include individuals well along in the grief process willing to participate in discussions with those more recently traumatized by loss. The long-term efficacy of these groups is well established, and they provide benefits even to those who are several months or years away from a tragic event.

Vignette

Dr. C was stunned by the news of his schizophrenic patient's suicide on the inpatient unit the night before he was scheduled to be discharged. Dr. C had asked about suicide daily, reviewed the notes for warning signs of self-harm, gone over the patient's safety plan, confirmed with the family their concurrence with the discharge and follow-up arrangements, and documented everything in standardized templates. The family's angry and accusatory response to the news left him shaken and uncertain. Reviewing the case repeatedly in his mind, Dr. C focused on the patient's paucity of speech throughout his stay as evidence of guarding and concluded that he had made a grave error in not recognizing this obvious sign of impending danger.

With great remorse, he acknowledged at the staff debriefing his failure to perceive the patient's suicidality. Others' emotions were intense, but most comments focused on their concern for the patient and grief at not being able to do more in his care. Dr. C came away from the meeting feeling relief that he was not blamed by the staff, but his confidence was not restored, and over the next few weeks, he continued to feel guilt and had difficulty making clinical decisions. Finally, a nurse took him aside and said simply, "You are being too hard on yourself; you are a good doctor, and we trust you." Dr. C was astonished by the relief that gave him.

Mortality and Morbidity Conferences

In the course of systems-based practice and improvement, the opportunity to learn from bad outcomes is a high priority, and there should be a mechanism to share the findings of the adverse event review with other clinicians. Several mechanisms to do this are available, the most common of which is the formal mortality and morbidity conference. The primary purpose of this conference is to formally present the case to a larger group of clinicians, typically the entire department, to allow them to learn from and share insights about the event. During this process, several other desirable outcomes may be achieved, including clarification of the facts of the case, suppression of rumors and misinformation, broadening of peer support, and creation of a sense of finality about the review process.

The usual format for the conference is to begin with a formal presentation of the case, generally culminating in the adverse event that triggered the review. The presentation may be limited to the objective facts of the case, such as the dates of events or the content of clinical notes. The presentation also may include additional explanatory information, such as the basis on which key decisions were made. Ideally, this would be clear from the medical record, but its absence is one of the most common deficiencies in clinical documentation.

In most instances, the case will be presented by the clinician most directly responsible for the care of the patient. In teaching centers, this may be a trainee, in which case the supervisor needs to be present and engaged in the conference. There are two major advantages to the primary clinician making the initial presentation. The first is to provide the most intimate knowledge of the course of treatment and condition of the patient as events unfolded. The second is to allow the primary clinician to confront the distress that invariably accompanies a bad outcome.

After a review of the facts of the case, several assigned discussants may take a few minutes to highlight pertinent issues, point out lesser-known facts relevant to the case, give different perspectives, confront misconceptions, share insights from their subspecialties, emphasize important teaching points, and highlight the key lessons of the event. Discussants may appropriately include the clinical supervisor for the case, subspecialists with expertise in critical areas, or other experienced clinicians who have handled similar cases. Senior clinicians who have experienced similar bad outcomes may be especially effective at sharing insights and support. Discussants establish and maintain the direction and limits of the discussion to ensure that it remains realistic and constructive.

Finally, there is an opportunity for open comment, questions, and discussion. It is critical that the atmosphere for this activity be appropriately managed to ensure that it is focused on the objectives of shared understanding and insights rather than judgment and blame. The goal is that everyone present emerges as a better clinician, armed with the benefit of this extreme experience, and that systems of care be improved by an understanding of where failures may have occurred.

These presentations have a confessional quality, an opportunity to share the ambiguity of information that was available, the uncertainty of decisions, and the focus of second-guessing and guilt that the case triggered. Consequently, trainees or junior clinicians view the activity with dread and terror. Most emerge, however, feeling exoneration and support. No one would advocate for an adverse event to occur, but if it does, it is of most benefit during residency or early career, when uncertainty about one's clinical skills and professional reputation makes one most vulnerable.

Vignette

Dr. D learned of her patient's suicide after an emergency department evaluation almost as an afterthought from a social worker who had called the family to check on how the patient was doing and was told of her death by overdose. She had been taken to another hospital for treatment, and no one had notified the previous providers. The case was designated a sentinel event because it had occurred so soon after her emergency department visit. Dr. D found the sentinel event review process painful and threatening, because she was asked innumerable questions about her thinking and decision-making and received no feedback from the institutional reviewers.

The patient, a young woman, made frequent visits to the emergency department with superficial cuts and transient suicidal ideation, usually in response to interpersonal tumult and her intense emotional reactions. Dr. D had declined to admit her but allowed her ample time to reconstitute in the psychiatric emergency department, assessed her suicidality carefully, checked in with her outpatient care providers, and arranged for the social work staff to call her after she got home. She privately recognized, however, that she had made a decision not to admit her even before beginning the evaluation, a fact she had been loath to acknowledge to anyone else. She dreaded having to present the case later at a departmental mortality and morbidity conference and agonized over the judgment she believed would be passed on her.

As she told the patient's story and the context in which it occurred, however, Dr. D was surprised by the understanding and support of those at the conference, so much so that she found herself sharing the secret that she believed had blinded her judgment. Far from receiving it with condemnation, the feedback she was given validated her decision, pointing out the patient's long pattern of unproductive admissions and the unpredictability of chaotic events in her life, one of which had immediately preceded her overdose. The conference proved to be more healing than traumatic and provided a public exoneration Dr. D had not expected.

Conclusion

Adverse events are a reality of medical care in every specialty, especially in the high-acuity settings of the hospital. Psychiatrists are especially vulnerable to the negative consequences of these events because of unrealistic expectations of institutions, families, and themselves and because of the nature of the working relationships that the profession demands. It is important to learn from every bad outcome and to honestly and systematically examine the care that was provided to find points for improvement. It is equally important to recognize the limitations of the field and not burden individuals or systems with onerous and unproductive measures. Finally, it is critical to ensure that supports are in place to assist clinicians with the difficult task of dealing with the loss of a patient to suicide or another unfavorable outcome.

KEY POINTS

- Adverse events are a reality of clinical care, especially in the high-acuity settings of the hospital.

- A system to report and review adverse events should be readily available to all medical center personnel, along with an established protocol for how to respond to those reports.

- Every adverse event should be reviewed, either formally or informally, depending on the nature and severity of the incident, to establish the facts of the case and identify potential areas for improvement in the system of care at the level of individual clinicians, teams, services, or the larger institution.

- Root cause analysis is a procedure to identify the fundamental issues leading to an unfavorable outcome in the hope that specific measures can be implemented to reduce the risk of future events.

- Medical errors differ from incidents involving flawed systems of practice and unpredictable or unpreventable events in that they involve a failure to follow established guidelines or standards of care.

- Reviews of adverse events, including mortality and morbidity conferences, serve both educational and administrative functions, allowing all clinicians to benefit vicariously from rare events and leaders to consider action plans when appropriate.

- Emotional, administrative, and legal support for all individuals involved in adverse events is critical to ensure the well-being of clinicians and other staff and the integrity of the institution.

Index

*Page numbers printed in **boldface** type refer to tables.*